POST-TRAUMATIC
NEUROSIS

POST-TRAUMATIC NEUROSIS

From Railway Spine to the Whiplash

Michael R. Trimble
Consultant Physician in Neuropsychiatry
and Senior Lecturer in Behavioural Neurology
The National Hospitals for Nervous Diseases
Queen Square, London WC1, England.

A Wiley Medical Publication

JOHN WILEY & SONS
Chichester · New York · Brisbane · Toronto

Copyright © 1981 by John Wiley & Sons Ltd.

British Library Cataloguing in Publication Data:

Trimble, Michael R.
   Post-traumatic neurosis.
   1. Traumatology
   I. Title
   617'.21   RD131

ISBN 0 471 09975 9

Typeset by Computacomp (UK) Ltd, Fort William, Scotland
Printed in The United States of America

For Jenifer—my compensation

Contents

Acknowledgements

I wish to thank Dr William Gooddy for the encouragement he gave me to continue writing this book, and for his many helpful comments on the completed manuscript. I am also indebted to my close friend and colleague Dr R. T. C. Pratt for reading and discussing the text, and for originally supporting my idea to tackle this difficult subject. In addition, I am grateful to others who have commented on various aspects of the manuscript, including Dr Jenifer Wilson-Barnett and Mr Charles Pugh. As always I am extremely grateful to Marge Zietsman for preparing and typing the manuscript, without whom none of this would be possible.

Introduction

J.R., a 55 year-old man from North London, led a relatively uneventful life until one day while at work a steel sling fell on to his head from the jib of a crane some 50 feet above him. The object weighed about 10 lb and the protective helmet that he was wearing at the time was knocked off by it. His own comments on the accident were: 'I don't know what happened, I was dazed.' He lost recall for the second or two before the accident and was unable to remember the next ten minutes of his life.

He was taken to hospital and examined and was then sent home, but according to his wife was 'pale and trembling'. He was sent to bed and stayed there for 24 hours, subsequently developing headaches, and when trying to get out of bed noted he had difficulty in balancing. His general practitioner saw him and confined him to bed where he stayed for several days complaining of headaches, giddiness, and loss of balance.

Two to three weeks later he tried to return to work but was unable to do so because of continuing symptoms. He was assessed at this time by a consultant in hospital who noted some pain in his neck and some weakness of his right arm, but on clinical examination did not find any detectable abnormalities. When his problems were still present a few weeks later he was taken into hospital and was further examined, although again with negative results.

As time passed he developed sudden and unexpected blackouts, and in addition a trembling of his right hand. Return to work became impossible on account of his continuing difficulties, and he subsequently developed sensations of anxiety and depression. His wife had to look after him, and she commented that he was a completely changed man, altering from someone who had been 'marvellous around the house' and placid, to a moody, irritable, and withdrawn person. As a couple they rarely went out, conversation became limited, and their sexual activity ceased.

He was investigated by several consultants following the initiation of legal proceedings by his solicitor. Two psychiatrists attested that he had a good premorbid personality, that he had had a stable marital relationship, and that his symptoms were attributable to the accident. His general practitioner who had known him for 20 years said he was 'a hardworking and reliable man'. Over that time he had seen him on but few occasions, not being a regular attender for tranquillizers and sleeping pills. Work records from his place of work indicated that he had rarely taken time off and confirmed his reliability as an employee.

On the other hand, two other doctors interpreted events rather differently. Both thought that he had received only a trivial blow to the head and were unable to determine any 'physical abnormalities'. They noted inconsistencies in his history, and during their examinations of him felt that the signs that he presented were incompatible with any known neurological illness. His paresis was referred to as 'a frank hysterical weakness' and his behaviour as 'a very histrionic display'. The two consultants expressed the opinion that he was a malingerer, one confidently asserting 'that he must be aware that his complaints are without genuine foundation'.

In the light of these conflicting medical opinions and the continued disability which the patient complained of, the date for the court hearing came nearer. The trial never went ahead however, a settlement of £30,000 being arranged between the insurance company involved and the plaintiff's solicitors.

This case history, with its substantial financial outcome, will have a familiar ring to those who deal with medico-legal compensation issues, and on reading it no doubt individuals will immediately be drawn to one of two feelings. The first of these, associated perhaps with a sense of indignation, would lead the reader to murmur in agreement with one of the opinions expressed, 'malingerer', with a feeling that Mr R had been extremely lucky to make off with a cool £30,000. An alternative feeling may be evoked in others however, possibly associated with the same sense of indignation, leading to comments that the case was 'typical' for post-traumatic neurosis, and that anybody who suggested the patient was a malingerer was merely reflecting insurance company views based on ill-founded evidence.

Readers not directly involved with these problems may wonder how this case could lead to such a conflict of views, and why such a fuss should be made over psychiatric symptomatology. The answer they would be given is simple—money. Thus, post-traumatic illness, especially but not always where negligence can be shown to have occurred leading to an accident, is compensatable. Someone has to pay, and in many cases this is insurance companies. Perhaps not unnaturally they seek to pay as little in settlement of claims as possible, and therefore have litigants examined by doctors of their own choice. In many situations there is little dispute about the amount that should be paid. Loss of an arm, leg, or an eye, are objectively noted, and from previous precedents the approximate amount of compensation awarded in the courts is easily assessed. However, when the patient's complaints are subjective and not easily verified by objective means, then their 'reality' becomes arguable, and such is the case with patients presenting with post-traumatic neurosis, the majority of the symptoms of which are entirely subjective. In many of these cases patients are told that, at the best they imagine their symptoms, and if they would pull up their socks they could do better. At worst, they are told they are malingering—falsifying their disability for financial gain. If this can be proven, and if the patient as a witness can be discredited, then the insurance company bill will be light.

However, many patients or those representing them also have physicians who give independent reports about their disability. These often stand in marked contrast to those of insurance company-based physicians, fully acknowledging the severity of post-traumatic neurotic symptoms, and implying that they are worthy of compensation. If and when these cases get to court, the various medical reports are presented, their discrepancies noted, and the legal machinery sets about deciding from the legal point of view what the outcome should be.

Debates over 'genuineness' of post-traumatic neurotic symptoms, and indeed the relationship of any symptoms to an accident, have continued for well over a century, and at the present time represent the veneer of a multimillion-pound enterprise involving insurance companies, government departments, unions, physicians, barristers, solicitors, social workers, and patients. Many doctors in the course of their practice come across these issues, and are asked to produce reports about patients, some of whom are not unlike Mr R. Surprisingly, very few studies have been carried out in this field and the literature available is full of opinion and devoid of facts. The dichotomy introduced above permeates these opinions, and the two sides are well represented from the early work in the late nineteenth century to the present day.

In this text I have attempted to review the available literature on the subject of post-traumatic neurosis, especially noting the dominant views that have been held at any one point in time, and which have changed with the passage of history. The debates really began in the 1860s with the writings of John Eric Erichsen on 'Concussion of the Spine' (see Chapter 1 references). His views crystallized contemporary thinking, which essentially stated that post-traumatic symptoms of a variety of kinds, including neurotic ones, were based in somatic damage. However, this view was soon to be challenged by Dr Page, another well-respected surgeon of the times, who introduced the concept of 'nervous shock' to explain the symptoms that patients presented with after accidents. All this occurred at a time when views regarding the aetiology of neuropsychiatric illness were altering, and concepts such as functional disorders and hysteria were changing their meaning as authors such as Charcot, Janet, and Freud put forward their ideas. These are briefly discussed in the text, as is the growing split between neurology and psychiatry which occurred around that time. As a consequence of this, post-traumatic neurotic symptoms became viewed as 'psychological' and their possible association with neurological damage minimized. The separation between psychiatry and neurology, between 'psychological' and 'neurological' disorders, is to some extent reflected in the dichotomy of views expressed regarding the cause of post-traumatic neurotic symptoms.

The literature in this field up to the present day is reviewed but in view of the paucity of data only a few hard conclusions can be reached. Some attempt at synthesis of views is made in the final chapter. Doubtless many will disagree with this, although I hope that readers will at least be stimulated to think further about these difficult issues, and some perhaps provoked to doing research to answer many of the unanswered questions.

CHAPTER 1

The Beginning—Railway Spine

In 1766 Dr Maty recorded in detail the case of Count de Lordat. Entitled 'A palsy occasioned by a fall attended with uncommon symptoms', it recounts how the Count, a French officer of 'great rank and much merit', overturned his carriage while on his way to join his regiment in 1761. 'His head pitched against the top of the coach; his neck was twisted from left to right; his left shoulder, arm and hand were much bruised.' He had few immediate problems from the injury, and was able to walk to the next town for assistance and to continue his journey as intended. He 'went through the fatigues of the campaign, which was a very trying one' but then, some six months after his accident, 'began to find an impediment to the utterance of words, and his left arm appeared to be weaker'. He underwent medical treatment which included bleeding, and returned to his regiment to undertake a second campaign. However by the end of it he had further difficulty in speaking, his left arm was even weaker, and he was forced to leave the army and return to Paris. Some three and half years after the accident, and following many consultations with physicians, his left arm 'withered more and more and the Count could hardly utter a few words'. Dr Maty reported:

'A more melancholy object I never beheld. The patient, naturally a handsome, middle-aged, sanguine man, of a cheerful disposition and an active mind, appeared much emaciated, stooping and dejected. He walked with a cane but with much difficulty and in a tottering manner. By this time it seems his left hand and arm were paralysed but also his right was somewhat benumbed, and he could scarcely lift it to his head.'

His saliva dribbled away; he could only utter monosyllables and 'these came out, after much struggling in a violent expiration and with a low tone and indistinct articulation'. We are also told that his senses and the powers of his mind were unaffected. The unfortunate Count died in March 1765, nearly four years after his accident, and a post-mortem examination was carried out. The 'pia mater of the brain was found "full of blood and lymph" and towards the falx there were some marks of suppuration. The medulla oblongata was said to be greatly enlarged and the membranes of the spinal cord were "greatly thickened and very tough".' Dr Maty concluded: 'From these appearances we were at no loss to fix the cause of the general palsy in the alterations of the medulla spinalis and oblongata.' The cause of these changes was related to the accident, and particularly to the twisting of the Count's neck during his fall (quoted by Erichsen, 1882).

The above case, recorded almost 60 years before the first railway was opened in this country, provides an example of the idea that injury, no matter how trivial it seems when it occurs, may provoke neurological illness which becomes apparent at some time in the future. Physicians of Dr Maty's era and before recognized this. Thus Sir Benjamin Brodie (1837), in a paper on injuries of the spinal cord wrote:

'The minute organisation of the spinal cord may suffer from a blow inflicted upon the spine, even where there is neither fracture or dislocation, and where the investing membranes do not appear to participate in any way in the effects of the injury. . . . In such cases if there be an opportunity of examining the spinal cord at a very early period after the accident has occurred, the central part of it is found to be softer than natural, its fibrous appearance being lost in that of semi-fluid substance. If the patient survives for a longer period, the alteration of structure is perceptible in the whole diameter of the cord, and occupies from one to two inches, or even more, of its length; and at a still later period it has often proceeded so far as to terminate in its complete dissolution. This disorganisation, softening, and final dissolution of the spinal cord is the most common consequence of injuries of the spine, and the dangerous symptoms which follow these accidents are, in the majority of cases, to be attributed to it.'

He went on to state categorically that 'the effect of a violent concussion is at once to impair and even to destroy the function of the spinal cord, sometimes even causing the patient's death in the course of a few hours'. The damage he felt was not the result of inflammation, but was often due to 'spasmodic affection of the muscles . . .' or 'pressure of extravasated blood', and the paper implied that 'disorganisation and dissolution of the cord' were the result of 'concussion'. He held similar views about the nature of symptoms following injuries to the brain. We were not justified, he felt, in assuming that as no changes were seen at post-mortem in cases of concussion of the brain, that there was therefore no organic injury.

'There may be changes and alterations in it which our senses are incapable of detecting. . . . These remarks are not less applicable to concussion of the spinal cord than they are to those of concussion of the brain. We cannot doubt that the nature of the injury is the same in both of them.'

Abercrombie (1828), in an apparently well-known textbook of the time, also commented that 'a severe blow to the spine frequently occasions an immediate loss of power in the parts below the seat of the injury without producing either fracture or dislocation of the vertebrae'. He quoted the case of a 54 year-old man who was temporarily paralysed after an accident in which he fell from a tree, but recovered with only a 'peculiar feeling of numbness, which was confined to the upper part of the left foot'. Some four years later, he developed an increased area of numbness, pain in the lower back, and paresis of the right leg, and ten years after the accident was paraplegic and incontinent. Abercrombie considered the symptoms were due to a disorganization of the activity of the spinal cord as a result of the blow.
The surgeon Syme (1862) was of the same viewpoint:

'The spinal cord is liable to concussion from blows and falls . . . the symptoms of which are similar to those of concussion of the brain, inasmuch as they denote suspension of the functions usually exercised by this part of the nervous system. As these consist chiefly in conduction of the impressions producing sensation and voluntary motion, the patient loses more or less completely the feeling and power of moving in all the portions of the body which are supplied with nerves originating from the spinal cord below the part where it has suffered from external violence. The organ does not recover from this state of irritation as soon as the brain. . . . It is probable that the cause of this may be effusion of the serum, or blood, occurring in consequence of the injury, which, subsequently undergoing absorption, allows the usual actions to be restored.'

Similar ideas regarding the aetiology of post-traumatic symptoms were prevalent abroad, both in America and on the continent of Europe. Mayo wrote on 'concussion of the spinal marrow' in his *Outlines of Human Pathology* (Mayo, 1836). He quoted several cases of seemingly trivial injuries with apparent recovery, where severe clinical symptoms developed after a time. Lidell (1864)—a surgeon in charge of the Stanton General Hospital in Washington, DC wrote:

'Clinical observation entirely aside from any speculation founded upon physiological and pathological knowledge has abundantly attested the exceeding gravity of all mechanical lesions of the spine. . . . It happens not infrequently that a paralysis, more or less complete, especially of the lower extremeties, is produced by injury of the spine without the occurrence of fracture, or, indeed of any perceptible lesion of the spinal column or of the spinal marrow. The term concussion of the spinal cord has been employed to designate these cases, because of the analogy they are supposed to bear to concussion of the brain. In both alike, a more or less complete arrest of spinal function is produced, without any visible injury to the nerve tissue.'

Writing on the spinal cord he said: 'for its anatomical relations are such that but little force is required to separate it from its osseous case, and in this way the spinal cord may be compressed in a manner analogous to what happens to the brain when blood is extravasated from the middle meningeal artery, between the cranium and the encephalic dura mater.' Likewise, Boyer (1814) was of a similar opinion, and wrote:

'Toute percussion violente portée sur l'épine, qu'elle produise ou non la fracture de quelqu'une des parties des vertèbres, ne donne pas ses effets à la colonne vertébrale. L'ébranlement se communique à la moelle de l'épine, et peut produire sur cet organe délient des mêmes effets que sur le cerveau. Ces effets sont beaucoup plus considérables. . . .'

It is clear that the general consensus of medical opinion around the midpoint of the last century was that 'concussion of the spinal cord' or 'spinal concussion' was a delineated entity in clinical literature, similar in its mechanism of production to concussion of the brain, and that the symptoms patients developed resulting from injury were due to organic lesions of the brain or spinal cord. A very influential work then appeared, which not only supported the above theories but had much influence on contemporary medico-legal thinking. John Eric Erichsen, Professor of Surgery at University College Hospital, London (see Plate 1), wrote a series of six lectures 'on certain obscure injuries of the nervous system commonly met with as the result of shocks to the body received in collisions on railways'. The lectures were published in 1866 and were incorporated into a book with eight new lectures and republished in 1875. The book was entitled *On Concussion of the Spine: nervous shock and other obscure injuries of the nervous system in their clinical and medico-legal aspects* (Erichsen, 1882). He made his intention clear on page one of his introduction, namely 'to direct attention to certain injuries of the spine that may arise from accidents that are often apparently slight, from shocks to the body generally, as well as from blows inflicted directly upon the back'. While he suggested that these kinds of injuries occurred in 'ordinary accidents of civic life—in falls, blows, horse and carriage accidents, injuries in gymnasiums, etc.' he commented that they occurred 'in none more frequently or with greater severity than in those which are sustained by persons who have been subjected to the violent shock of railway collision . . . injuries of the nervous system of the kind we are about to discuss have become of much practical importance from the great frequency of their occurrence consequent on the extension of railway traffic. . . .'

Although 'railways' in one form or another had been in use for at least 200 years, particularly in the haulage of goods from one place to another, the nineteenth century saw an expansion of this means of transport for passenger travel. The advent of steam engines, the use of iron rails rather than of wood, and the needs of industrial revolution led to the widespread development of a railway system, initially against much opposition. The Liverpool and Manchester Railway opened on September 15, 1830, ushering in the railway age, and with it inevitable railway accidents. The first accident occurred on the day of the opening. Halfway down the line some guests got off the train to look at the engine and one them, William Huskisson, MP for Liverpool, was fatally injured by the 'Rocket' running on an adjacent line. The opposers of the railways, in the light of this accident, were quick to point out the dangers of the system, but were soon quietened as the network of railway traffic grew and its usefulness became apparent. Six thousand miles of railway were built between 1836 and 1852. With more and more accidents, victims were examined and reported on by doctors, and Erichsen was one of the first to suggest that there may

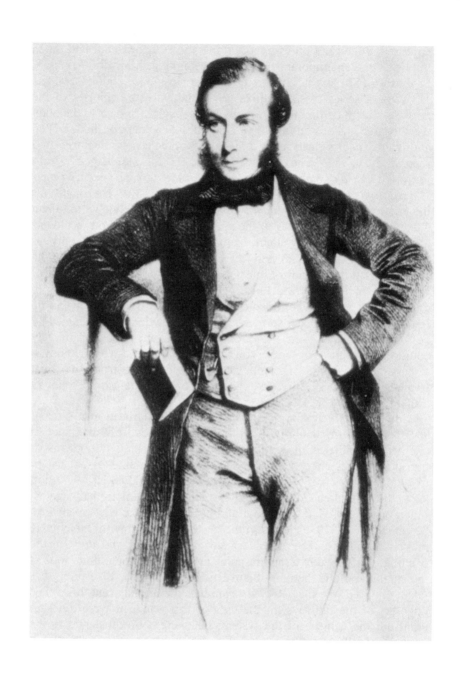

Plate 1 (a) John Eric Erichsen

ON

CONCUSSION OF THE SPINE

NERVOUS SHOCK

AND OTHER OBSCURE INJURIES OF THE NERVOUS SYSTEM

IN THEIR

CLINICAL AND MEDICO-LEGAL ASPECTS

BY

JOHN ERIC ERICHSEN, F.R.S.

SURGEON EXTRAORDINARY TO THE QUEEN; EMERITUS PROFESSOR OF CLINICAL
SURGERY IN UNIVERSITY COLLEGE, AND CONSULTING SURGEON TO
THE HOSPITAL; EX-PRESIDENT OF THE ROYAL COLLEGE OF
SURGEONS OF ENGLAND, AND OF THE ROYAL
MEDICAL AND CHIRURGICAL SOCIETY
ETC.

'Je raconte, je ne juge pas'—*Montaigne*

A NEW AND REVISED EDITION

LONDON

LONGMANS, GREEN, AND CO.

1882

have been something special about the sequelae of being involved in a railway accident.

When Erichsen was writing his book there was a considerable amount of information already available about the consequences of more severe injuries of the nervous system, but much less was known of the results of more minor ones. His task was not easy.

'There is indeed no class of cases in which medical men are now so frequently called upon to give evidence in the courts of law, as those which involve the many intricate questions that arise in actions for damages against railway companies for injuries of the nervous system, alleged to have been sustained by passengers in collisions; and there is no class of cases in which more discrepancy of surgical opinion may be elicited.'

He began by defining and supporting the concept of 'concussion of the spine'. This term had been objected to by some on the grounds that it was usual to speak of 'concussion of the brain' and not 'concussion of the head', and thus a better term for the spinal injury was really 'concussion of the cord'. Erichsen, however, felt that the spine was really a far more complicated structure than the head, and pointed out that injury of the spine not only involved the cord but also injury to bone, ligaments, and muscle which are an intricate part of the spine. Trauma to these accessories he felt were responsible for some of the most severe and persistent symptoms of injury. He then defined 'concussion of the spine':

It may be stated that this phrase is generally adopted . . . to indicate a certain state of the spinal cord occasioned by external violence; a state that is independent of, and usually, but not necessarily, uncomplicated by any obvious lesion of the vertebral column, such as its fracture or dislocation—a condition that is supposed to depend upon a shake or a jar received by the cord, in consequence of which its intimate organic structure may be more or less deranged, and by which its functions are certainly greatly disturbed, so that various symptoms indicative of loss or modification of innervation are immediately or remotely induced.'

He speculated on the nature of the underlying pathology:

'The primary effects of these concussions or commotions of the spinal cord are probably due to molecular changes in its structure.

The secondary are mostly of an inflammatory character, or are dependent on retrogressive organic changes, such as softening, etc., consequent on interference with its nutrition.'

With this initial commitment he thus clearly identified with the organic view which characterized thought at this time. He warned that the condition could start at an early age and reported: 'I have even known the slapping of the back of a new-born infant to lead it to breathe to develop into caries of the spine.'

The book contained 53 case histories of patients who had received injuries of a wide variety. The outcome of the cases varied from recovery to death, and not all were due to direct injury of the brain or spinal cord. His 'Case 50' is tabulated as 'Crush of Finger—Tetanic Spasms—Progressive Disease of the Nervous System—Death'. This interesting case is reproduced in full with its conclusions.

'A gentleman, aged 60, in good health, when travelling to the City on March 24th, 1866, on one of the suburban lines of railway had one of his fingers crushed between the door and its frame on the hinge side. The accident gave rise to great pain, and to some loss of blood. The sufferer returned home faint and exhausted with the shock. He was seen and the finger dressed by Dr Wightman, who found there had been considerable contusion and laceration of its extremity, but that the bones were uninjured. The wound healed slowly but satisfactorily, yet the patient, who was in robust health and weighed about twenty stone at the time of the accident lost flesh, became weak, and never seemed completely to rally from the shock that he had sustained. In the course of a month, twitchings, shooting pains, and cramps in the arm, somewhat resembling slight tetanic spasms, developed themselves. On April 29 he had a slight fit. This was followed by numbness, sensations of pins and needles in the hand and arm, twitchings of the face; a sense of weariness and of weakness, and although he had previously to the accident been a strong man, he was now unable to undergo even slight exertion without much feeling of fatigue. He, however, returned to his business as a house agent, and for six months continued it intermittently. He was then obliged to relinquish it, grew slowly and gradually worse, and eventually died, with symptoms of cerebral softening on September 13th, 1867. Previously to this he had been seen by Mr. Le Gros Clark, and a consultation had been arranged on the day of his death, which was sudden. The question arose as to how far these symptoms were connected with the accident, and after a careful review of all the circumstances of the case, we came to the opinion that the injury received in the hand was the exciting cause of the affection of the nervous system which ultimately resulted in his death.'

Erichsen enlightened us as to the thought processes underlying his decision.

'The circumstances that mainly led to this conclusion were the following: That up to the time of the accident the patient had been in robust health; that the injury was immediately followed by severe and prolonged nervous shock, and by signs of local nervous irritation of the arm; that he never subsequently recovered from these symptoms, which were continuous, without a break, and though at times somewhat fluctuating, were, upon the whole, slowly progressive, the disease which originated in the injury having, in point of fact, an uninterrupted history from its origin to its fatal termination; that the hand and arm of the injured wrist were the primary seats of the local disease which spread upwards to the nervous centres; and that death resulted from cerebral disease which presented all the signs of softening of the brain.'

This example is important not only because of the consequences, in that we are told the patient's widow brought a legal action against the company and 'obtained a verdict', but because it highlights two of the recurrent themes of Erichsen's book. First, the implication that organic lesions follow from relatively mild trauma—essentially the message conveyed in the other cases reported. Second, the case involved injury on a railway train—even though it was not consequent upon an actual railway accident. Although Erichsen made the point that the term 'railway spine' was an 'absurd appellation' in that similar events were seen following all varieties of accidents, and had been described many years before the first railway was opened, he was not altogether impartial in his references to railways. Thus 'the peculiarities of these obscure injuries of the nervous system caused by railway shocks is sufficiently great, however, to warrant us in grouping them together, and considering them as a whole in a separate chapter of a great book of surgery'. While he objected to the term 'railway spine', seven of his case histories are tabulated as 'railway shock' and two 'railway collision'. There were, he said, several things which appeared noteworthy about railway accidents, including his observation that persons injured in any one accident presented with very similar symptoms.

'This may be accounted for, to some extent at least, and in some cases, though certainly not in all, by the severity of the collision and the resulting intensity of the shock, varying in different accidents according to the rapidity with which the train is travelling at the moment of collision, or the force with which it is run into from behind.'

He elaborated further on the mechanism of the railway injuries:

'I have often remarked that in railway accidents those passengers suffer most seriously from concussion of the nervous system who sit with their backs turned towards the end of the train which is struck. Thus when a train runs into an obstruction on the line, those who are sitting with their backs to the engine will probably suffer most; whilst if a train is run into from behind, those who are facing the engine will most frequently be the greatest sufferers. The explanation of this fact appears to me as follows. When a train runs into a stationary impediment, its momentum is suddenly arrested, whilst that of the passengers still continues. Those who are facing the engine are in the first instance thrown suddenly and violently forwards off their seats against the opposite side of the compartment, hence they will frequently be found to be cut about the head and face, and more especially across the knees and legs, by coming in contact with the edge of the opposite seats. They then rebound, and in the rebound may sustain that concussion of the spine which they escaped in the first shock. Those, on the other hand, who are sitting with their backs to the engine, being carried backwards when the momentum of the carriage is suddenly arrested are struck at once; and if travelling rapidly, are jerked violently against the back of their seats, and thus suffer in the first instance and by the first shock from concussion of the spine. The force with which they strike the partition between the compartments with their shoulders or loins is greatly augmented by their opposite fellow-travellers being thrown upon them. In the oscillation and to-and-fro movement to which the carriage is subjected they are apt to be thrown forwards, and rebounding to be struck again about the posterior part of the body. They are more helpless than those who are facing the engine, who frequently have time to stretch out their hands in order to save themselves, or to clutch hold of the sides of the carriage when in the act of being thrown forwards. When a carriage is run into from behind, the reverse of this takes place, and the carriage is driven, as it were, against those passengers who have got their backs turned towards the hind part of the train. In the violent oscillations that take place a passenger is thrown backwards and forwards by a kind of shuttlecock action, and frequently coming in contact with others on the opposite side, may become seriously injured, especially by contusions about the head. The oscillations to which the body is subjected in these accidents are chiefly felt in those parts of the vertebral column that admit of most movement, viz. at the junction of the head and neck, of the neck and shoulders, and of the trunk and pelvis. Hence it is that the spine so frequently becomes strained and injured in these regions by railway injuries.'

In addition to the more severe forms of illness that followed injury to the head and spine, Erichsen also devoted a chapter to 'sprains, twists and wrenches of the spine'. Such injuries he felt were commoner than the former, nevertheless they were no less dangerous to the individual. 'They may be followed by every possible kind of mischief . . . which appears to be expended on the spine itself independently of its contents, which escape uninjured.' One mechanism whereby he suggested this occurred is reminiscent of the so-called 'whiplash injury'.

'In railway collisions, when a person is violently and suddenly jolted from one side of the carriage to the other, the head is frequently forcibly thrown forwards and backwards, moving as it were by its own weight, the patient having momentarily lost control over the muscular structures of the neck. . . .'

He recounted case histories of such strains which had resulted in serious morbidity and in one case proved fatal.

Erichsen, like observers before and after him, was struck by the disproportion that occurred between an apparently minor accident and the severe consequences. Even more perplexing perhaps was that the symptoms of 'spinal concussion' were rarely seen when there had been serious injury to the limbs, unless the spine itself had been struck directly.

'It would appear as if the violence of the shock expended itself in

17

the production of the fracture or the dislocation, and that a jar of
the more delicate nervous structure is thus avoided.'

He explained this further by using an analogy a watch-maker had told
him. When a watch falls to the ground, '. . . if the glass was broken, the
works were rarely damaged; if the glass escapes unbroken, the jar of
the fall will usually be found to have stopped the movement'.
He expressed uncertainty as to the actual pathogenesis of the
concussion but of the consequences he had no doubt.

'But whatever may be the nature of the primary change that is
produced in the spinal cord by a concussion, the secondary effects
are clearly of an inflammatory character, and are identical with
those phenomena that have been described by Oliver,
Abercrombie, and others, as dependent on chronic meningitis of
the cord and sub-acute myelitis.'

Lamenting the lack of post-mortem material, and confessing his own
lack of such material, he did report one case where a post-mortem had
been carried out. He quoted from the *Transactions of the Pathological
Society* by Lockhart Clarke. The patient, a 52 year-old man, died three
and a half years after a railway accident in which he suffered no
external sign of injury. On examination 'traces of chronic inflammation
were found in the arachnoid and cortical substance of the brain. The
spinal meninges were greatly congested and exudative matter had been
deposited upon the surface of the cord . . .'. This case he said afforded
evidence of the changes that take place in the cord under the influence
of 'concussion of the spine' from a railway accident.
A second important mechanism in the production of symptoms
invoked by Erichsen was by the process of spinal anaemia. This
condition was long known to physicians as a cause of a disease called
'spinal irritability' and which could have graver consequences resulting
in paralysis. Spinal anaemia was said by Erichsen to occur most often
in young people under the age of 35, especially women. Since the
disease was never fatal there was no post-mortem material available for
examination, and the possible explanation as to how the anaemia was
brought about was as follows.

'Whether it is by a concussion or vibratory jar in consequence of
which its molecular condition is so disturbed that its functions
become for a time perverted or suspended, or whether, as may not
improbably be the case, the primary lesion has been inflicted upon

the sympathetic system of nerves, in consequence of which the vascular supply to the cord may have become interfered with, and the symptoms that have just been described have directly resulted from a diminution of arterial blood transmitted to it, as the result of the disturbance of the vasomotor action of the sympathetic is uncertain.'

Erichsen's work was extremely influential and attracted much attention both in Europe and in the United States. Several writers, all experienced in the management of medico-legal cases of accidents, publishing within seven years of the appearance of the expanded version of Erichsen's book, made important contributions to the subject. For example, Leyden (1875) devoted a chapter of his book to the disorders of the spinal cord, and considered railway injuries in particular. He described small lesions and haemorrhages in the substance of the cord at post-mortem in some patients, and commented:

'The cases are very prone, where they have endured for a time without improvement, to assume an imitative character, leading to difficult and sometimes dangerous forms of myelitis, with its multiform bad consequences.'

He like Erichsen, was subscribing to the view not only that even minor injuries may be followed by most severe symptoms, but also that the symptoms produced were the consequence of progressive neurological disease. The term 'spinal concussion' actually was referred to eponymously as 'Erichsen's disease' popularized in 1889 by Clevenger, an American physician. He published a book with the title *Spinal Concussion: surgically considered as a cause of spinal injury, and neurologically restricted to a certain symptom group, for which is suggested the designation Erichsen's disease as one form of the traumatic neuroses* (Clevenger, 1889). In it he supported Erichsen's views, and put forward evidence that the symptoms noted were due to abnormalities of the sympathetic nervous system arising out of the accident.

The disorder and its accompanying pathology were seized upon by litigants and their friends. They 'were appraised of clinical and pathological possibilities that were before this undreamed of . . . Erichsen's little volume became a guide book that might lead the dishonest plaintiff, if he felt so disposed, to set out upon a broad road of imposture and dissimulation with the expectation of getting a heavy

Spinal Concussion:

*SURGICALLY CONSIDERED AS A CAUSE OF SPINAL IN-
JURY, AND NEUROLOGICALLY RESTRICTED TO
A CERTAIN SYMPTOM GROUP, FOR WHICH
IS SUGGESTED THE DESIGNATION*

ERICHSEN'S DISEASE,

AS ONE FORM OF THE TRAUMATIC NEUROSES.

BY

S. V. CLEVENGER, M.D.,

CONSULTING PHYSICIAN REESE AND ALEXIAN HOSPITALS; LATE PATHOLOGIST COUNTY INSANE ASYLUM,
CHICAGO; MEMBER OF NUMEROUS AMERICAN SCIENTIFIC AND MEDICAL SOCIETIES; COLLABORATOR
AMERICAN NATURALIST, ALIENIST AND NEUROLOGIST, JOURNAL OF NEUROLOGY AND
PSYCHIATRY, JOURNAL OF NERVOUS AND MENTAL DISEASES; AUTHOR OF "COM-
PARATIVE PHYSIOLOGY AND PSYCHOLOGY," "ARTISTIC ANATOMY," ETC.

WITH THIRTY WOOD-ENGRAVINGS.

With the Compliments of the author
Febry 12 90

PHILADELPHIA AND LONDON:
F. A. DAVIS, PUBLISHER,
1889.

20

verdict' (Hamilton, 1906). Few cases it seems were taken to court without the book appearing and being quoted. The tone of litigation claims changed. In the nineteenth century and before, legal cases involved with personal injury were mainly to do with material injuries, such as loss of a limb or an eye, where objective evidence was unmistakable and quantifiable. With the advent of 'concussion of the spine' the situation changed, and the concept that the injured were victims of at best 'shock' and at worst spinal anaemia or meningitis became prevalent.

References

Abercrombie, J. (1828) *Diseases of the Brain and Spinal Cord.* 4th Edition, London, Longmans.
Boyer, A. (1814) *Maladies Chirurgicales.* Cinquième édition, Paris, Migneret.
Brodie, B. (1837) *Injuries to the Spinal Cord. Medico-Chirurgical Transactions* **20,** 118.
Clevenger, S. V. (1889) *Spinal Concussion.* F. A. Davis, London.
Erichsen, J. E. (1882) *On Concussion of the Spine: nervous shock and other obscure injuries of the nervous system in their clinical and medico-legal aspects.* Longmans, Green & Co., London.
Hamilton, A. M. (1906) *Railway and other Accidents.* Baillière, Tindall and Co., London.
Leyden, E. (1875) *Klinik der Rückenmarkskrankheiten,* Band II, Berlin.
Lidell, J. A. (1864) On injuries of the spine including concussion of the spinal cord. *American Journal of the Medical Sciences* **48,** 305.
Mayo, H. (1836) *Outlines of Human Pathology.* London, Burgess and Hill.
Syme, J. (1862) *Observations on Clinical Surgery.* 2nd Edition. Edinburgh.

CHAPTER 2

An Alternative—The Contributions of Dr Page

In 1883 Herbert Page, surgeon to the London and North-West Railway, published a book entitled *Injuries of the Spine and Spinal Cord without apparent Mechanical Lesion* (Page, 1885). This was essentially a rebuttal of the ideas expressed by Erichsen. From the outset Page was critical of the latter's book, even as to its title. Concussion of the Spine Page felt was an indefinite expression, scientifically inaccurate and illogical. He castigated Erichsen for quoting the case of the Count de Lordat thus:

'A terrible case, forsooth, to be pointed out as "typical"; and typical of what? Of the whole class of injuries of the spine grouped together under the one common term 'concussion'. . . . Small wonder when a man gets a slight sprain of his vertebral column in the most trifling collision on a railway that, labouring under the belief he has received a "concussion of the spine", his anxiety should be needlessly great and prolonged if he learns that the result of the injury in this often-quoted case of the Count de Lordat is the typical result of such a "concussion of the spine" as he has himself received, even though he does not increase his risks of protracted illness by going through two campaigns. The dust of the unhappy Count must have undergone a "molecular disturbance" in its tomb when, in the very opening pages of the book, this painful history was transcribed as "typical of the whole class of injuries" grouped under the term "concussion of the spine".'

Page, quoting similar cases recorded by Sir Charles Bell, felt the

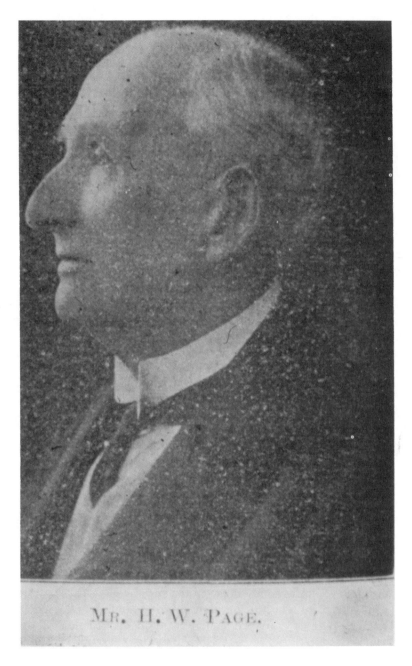

MR. H. W. PAGE.

Plate 3 (a)   Mr Herbert Page

INJURIES

OF THE

SPINE AND SPINAL CORD

WITHOUT APPARENT MECHANICAL LESION,

AND

NERVOUS SHOCK,

IN THEIR

SURGICAL AND MEDICO-LEGAL ASPECTS

BY

HERBERT W. PAGE, M.A., M.C. Cantab.,

FELLOW OF THE ROYAL COLLEGE OF SURGEONS OF ENGLAND;

SURGEON TO, AND LECTURER ON SURGERY AT, ST. MARY'S HOSPITAL   FORMERLY
SURGEON TO THE CUMBERLAND INFIRMARY

SECOND EDITION

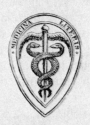

LONDON

J. & A. CHURCHILL

NEW BURLINGTON STREET

1885

injuries of the Count resulted probably from traumatic inflammation of the spinal membranes, although syphilis was a possible cause that could not be discounted. Page then discussed some of the other case histories recorded by Erichsen and attempted to discredit them. Having disassembled the latter's evidence Page was of the opinion that there were few or no facts to support the idea that the spinal cord suffered from 'concussion' in the absence of simultaneous injury to the spinal column. He wrote:

'used now to indicate this injury, and now that, here signifying the cause, there the effect, by a writer so distinguished as Mr Erichsen, it is little wonder that a wider application even has been given to the term, and that, as we shall see by and by, "concussion of the spine" is used almost indiscriminately both in and outside the medical profession to indicate the injuries which are received in collisions and which become the subject of medico-legal enquiry, although the spinal column and its contents have met with no damage at all. It appears to us nothing less than lamentable that Mr Erichsen should not have been more clear, more explicit, and less ambiguous in the case of phrases which he has employed.'

Another point on which he took Erichsen to task was the rarity of post-mortems. With all the thousands of people who were involved in railway collisions over the years, it was very surprising that there had been such a lack of post-mortem material. 'How is it,' Page wrote, 'that these diseases of the spinal cord are, if we mistake not, rarely or never seen in the special hospitals devoted to them, and that at such a hospital as the National Hospital for Epilepsy and Paralysis, in Queen Square, with its justly distinguished staff, they should be well-nigh unknown?'

Page detailed some 234 of his own cases. These he reported were unselected, but were all cases which related to collision. He recorded not only a brief sketch of the accidents, but also any data of legal settlement and date of follow-up.

Page introduced to his writings the concept of 'nervous shock', bringing to the debate a line of thought almost absent from the writings of Erichsen.

'Nervous shock in its varied manifestations is so common after railway collisions, and the symptoms thereof play so prominent a part in all cases which become the subject of medico-legal enquiry, whether they be real or feigned, that we are almost sure to meet with the symptoms of it associated with pains and points of tenderness along the vertebral spinous processes. . . . We cannot help thinking that it is this combination of the symptoms of general nervous prostration or shock and pains in the back, . . . which has laid the foundation of the views—erroneous views as we hold them to be—so largely entertained of the nature of these common injuries of the back received in railway collisions.'

Erichsen had taken little account of possible 'nervous' symptoms and, as noted in a later chapter, had little constructive to say on the possible nature and occurrence of hysteria after accidents. Page felt it was germane to consider the bones and ligaments that contribute to the structure of the spinal cord as a possible seat of symptoms, and that complaints arising from such structures could be severe, but felt they should receive 'no more import than they deserve', discounting to his readers the whole concept of 'railway spine'.

From his own cases Page was unable to find any case of subacute or chronic meningitis which followed railway injury, and he highlighted a diagnostic error of the supporters of 'railway spine'. While pain localized over one or more vertebrae was often quoted as evidence of spinal meningitis this clearly was incorrect. He quoted Gowers' textbook, *Diagnosis of Diseases of the Spinal Cord*, as authority that the symptoms—'the only symptoms'—which usually result from meningitis, 'are those which result from the involvement of the nerve roots in their passage through diseased membranes . . .'. Additionally he recognized that coincident disease such as syphilis may be present prior to the accident, and lead to the symptoms which later became associated with 'railway spine'.

'We have very carefully gone into, and we have endeavoured to meet with cases where there has been degeneration of the spinal cord as a remote consequence of spinal injury. Our enquiries have either been singularly unsuccessful . . . or we must admit that secondary and remote degeneration of the spinal cord in cases where there has been no definitive evidence of injury, is very rare indeed.'

As to Erichsen's suggestions that 'molecular disturbances' were in part responsible for the symptoms observed, Page was equally dogmatic.

'Molecular disturbance is not necessarily molecular disintegration or pathological change, and there is no evidence to show that molecular disturbance is in itself a grave condition, or likely to have evil results, unless there should have been at the time some well-marked pathological lesion.'

Page therefore was of the opinion that it was extremely rare for the spinal cord to be damaged in accidents when the spinal apparatus supporting the cord was undamaged. When damage to the spinal apparatus did occur, however, then there were accompanying unequivocal clinical signs and the outcome was more severe. In cases where there were undoubted signs and symptoms soon after the injury, which then cleared up, the pathology was probably haemorrhage which gradually reabsorbed, relieving any pressure that had built up.

Having thus discussed and dismissed so-called 'concussion of the spine', Page was then left with explaining the large number of patients who, after accident and trivial injury, presented with symptoms. He described the phenomenon of 'general nervous shock' and introduced the reader to the concept of 'functional disorders'.

'We use "shock to the nervous system" as a term applicable rather to the whole clinical circumstances of the case than to any one symptom which may be presented by the injured person . . . the course, history and general symptoms indicate some functional disturbance of the whole nervous balance or tone rather than structural damage to any organ of the body.'

He then defined what we now understand as surgical shock, as a consequence of more serious injury or blood loss, and continued as follows:

'Compare two cases of like injury, the one received by accident on a railway and the other by being knocked down and run over in the street, and the probabilities are great that the manifestations of shock will in the former case be more extreme than in the latter. And the difference lies in this, that in one case there is an element of great fear and alarm, which has perhaps been altogether absent from what may be called the less formidable and less terrible mode of accident . . . medical literature abounds with cases where the gravest disturbances of function, and even death or the annihilation of function, have been produced by fright and by fright alone. It is this same element of fear which in railway conditions has so large a share—in many cases the only share—in inducing immediate collapse, and in giving rise to those after-symptoms which may be almost as serious as, and are certainly far more troublesome than, those which we meet shortly after the accident has occurred.'

He was in no doubt about the horror of actually being involved in a railway accident, and unless the experience had actually happened to a person it would be difficult to conceive what it must have been like. Page quoted Mr Furneaux Jordan on the subject:

'The incidents of a railway accident contribute to form a combination of the most terrible circumstances which it is possible for the mind to conceive. The vastness of the destructive forces, the magnitude of the results, the imminent danger to the lives of numbers of human beings, and the hopelessness of escape from the danger, give rise to emotions which in themselves are quite sufficient to produce shock or even death itself . . .'

A perhaps better known description of what it is actually like to be in a railway accident, and some of its consequences, was recorded by Charles Dickens, whose accounts give some insight into the events that Page was describing. Dickens was in a railway accident at Staplehurst in Kent on June 9th, 1865. In a letter to Thomas Miller, four days after the affair he wrote:

'Two ladies were my fellow passengers, an old one and a young one. This is exactly what passed. You may judge from it the precise length of the suspense: suddenly we were off the rail, and beating the ground as the car of a half emptied balloon might. The old lady cried out "My God!" and the young one screamed. I caught hold of them both (the old lady sat opposite and the young one on my left) and said: "We can't help ourselves, but we can be quiet and composed. Pray don't cry out." The old lady immediately answered: "Thank you. Rely upon me. Upon my soul I will be quiet." We were all there tilted down together in the corner of the carriage and stopped. I said to them thereupon: "You may be sure nothing worse can happen. Our danger *must* be over. You will remain here without stirring, while I get out of the window." They both answered quite collectively "Yes" and I got out without the least notion of what had happened.'

In another letter Dickens commented:

'I was in the carriage that did not go over the bridge, but which caught on one side and hung suspended over the ruined parapet. I am shaken but not by that shock. Two or three hours' work afterwards among the dead and dying surrounded by terrific sights, render my hand unsteady.'

The shock that he referred to did not only have immediate effects on him, but the delayed consequences were also recorded. Some time after the accident he wrote:

'I am not quite right within, but believe it to be an effect of the railway shaking. There is no doubt of the fact that, after the Staplehurst experience, it tells more and more (railway shaking, that is) instead of, as one might have expected, less and less. . . .'

And later:

'I am curiously weak—weak as if I were recovering from a long illness . . . I begin to feel it more in my head. I sleep well and eat well; but I write half a dozen notes, and turn faint and sick,'

or

'I am getting right, though still low in pulse and very nervous. Driving in Rochester yesterday I felt more shaken than I have since the accident. I cannot bear railway travelling yet. A perfect conviction, against the senses, that the carriage is down on one side (and generally that is the left, and *not* the side on which the carriage in the accident really went over), comes upon me with anything like speed, and is inexpressibly distressing.' (Forster, 1969)

Page then, in complete contrast to Erichsen, introduced into his argument the concept of nervous shock, which was essentially psychological in origin.

'In these purely psychical causes lies, we believe, the explanation of the remarkable fact that after railway collisions the symptoms of general nervous shock are so common, and often so severe, in those who have received no bodily injury. . . .'

He is quite emphatic:

'The collapse from severe bodily injury is coincident with the injury itself, or with the immediate results of it, but when the shock is produced by purely mental causes the manifestations thereof may be delayed. . . .'

He emphasized that in assessing the consequences of railway collisions, due emphasis must be given to the alarm and nervous state as a cause of the patient's symptoms.

'We are inclined to think that sufficient importance has not hitherto been attached to it, and that many errors in diagnosis have been made because fright has not been considered of itself sufficient—as undoubtedly it is sufficient—to bring about the train of symptoms which we shall seek to describe.'

He not only drew a distinction between the physical injuries and the symptoms due to psychological causes, he also said the former manifest themselves in 'unmistakable signs'. Giving examples of cases which he felt demonstrated his second category of patients, he was at pains to point out that 'they are examples free, as we believe, from the taint of conscious exaggeration. . . .'

He was critical of the idea of 'anaemia of the cord' as a possible explanation of some of the symptoms he described in his patients, and called on the weighty evidence of Gowers and Erb to support him, essentially advising caution on the grounds of complete lack of confirmation. Thus one piece of evidence apparently often quoted in the courts as support for the presence of anaemia was the ophthalmological opinion. In that the blood vessels of the fundus can be seen and described, their state in victims of railway injuries was often supposed to show altered blood flow, indicative of either anaemia or hyperaemia of the nervous system. Page himself never found any lesion or pathological changes on such an examination except in cases where the eyeball itself had been injured. He quoted Gowers:

'The subject of the changes in the optic discs in spinal injuries has received a large amount of attention in consequence of the prominence which "railway cases" have given to this class of accident. In its scientific relations the subject has not escaped the sinister influence which litigation exercises on the investigation of facts, and there is no doubt that the pathological nature of many of the appearances described in these cases have been the result of an affection of the mind of the observer, rather than of the eye observed.'

The views of Page must have been welcomed by the legal counsels of railway companies, and presumably Mr Page's book, like that of Mr Erichsen before, was soon a familiar sight in courtroom trials. He was not alone in his opinions however and found support from writers both here and abroad. On Concussion of the Spine, Shaw (1870) commented 'the term concussion as applied to the spinal cord has obviously been derived from the supposed analogy between the injuries occurring to it and to its kindred organ the brain . . .'. However, the author pointed out this was false in that the surroundings of the two were entirely different. Unlike the brain, the spinal cord is surrounded by 'dampers', and it occupies the centre of a 'roomy chamber' at a considerable distance from the surrounding bony suprastructure. 'Even if the spine did vibrate there would be no connecting medium capable of conducting the vibrations to the cord.' He also said, echoing Page:

'When the body is jolted, jarred, and shaken in the violent manner described . . . the account would be incomplete if the influences of mental shock—that of fright and of witnessing appalling spectacles—were neglected. . . . On the whole it may be affirmed, that what is most wanted for the better understanding of those cases commonly known under the title of "concussion of the spine" is a greatly enlarged number of post-mortem examinations. Hitherto our experience has been derived almost wholly from litigated cases, deformed by contradictory statements and opinions; and the verdicts of juries have stood in the place of post-mortem reports.'

Le Gros Clark (1870) in Lectures on the Principles of Surgical Diagnosis also dealt with the problem in a similar way. While conceding there was a group of patients with symptoms which in spite of there being no evidence of a physical lesion; 'there must be organic change which is often progressive', he said;

. . . in others the morbid condition is evinced by deteriorated health and defective nerve energy; and in these probably the impaired health is due to the indirect influence exercised on the organs of assimilation, and a reactionary impression exerted on the nerve centres themselves. . . . . There is no immediate persistent incapacity, as in ordinary concussion from a blow to the head or spine; but a prolonged series of symptoms ensue, directly traceable to the shock, and often assuming a more aggravated character as time elapses.'

The *Boston Medical and Surgical Journal* in the 1880s carried a series of articles all bearing on the issue of 'so-called concussion of the spine', which supported Page's views. In 1881 the American, Hodges, attempted to make a more rational classification of the sequelae. Thus, whereas Erichsen had used the term 'spinal concussion' indiscriminately for cases which seemed to arise from 'organic damage' and 'functional change' of the nervous system, Hodges suggested the former should be clearly separated from the latter. Then organic changes could be diagnosed by their correct pathological name (e.g. meningitis), and their prognosis which is known can be accurately assessed and given. Putnam (1881), in a paper to the Boston Society for Medical Improvement, continuing these ideas, suggested that the cases described as due to functional disorder were capable of further classification. After duly acknowledging the 'special service which Mr Page has rendered', he made the point that some at least of the cases described were examples 'of that important neurosis which is called hysteria'. Although Erichsen had used the term hysteria, it is unclear exactly what he meant by it. As indicated in the next chapter this is largely due to the fact that the concept of hysteria was undergoing change at the end of the nineteenth century. However, when Putnam was writing, the works of Charcot and others who were involved in investigating hysteria were more widely known than when Erichsen described his cases. Indeed Putnam said of hysteria that it was 'a term which, thanks to the labours of Charcot and his pupils, has vastly outgrown its old and vague meaning, and is constantly acquiring a more precise and practical significance'.

Walton (1883) contributed further to the ideas of the time by suggesting that it was the brain, rather than the spinal cord, which was the main seat of injury in these accidents. Pointing out, as others had done, that the cord hangs suspended in a large cavity surrounded by loose tissue and fluid, he suggested it was less likely to suffer from the results of injury than the brain. The latter is not only heavier than the cord, but also lies in relatively intimate connection with its surrounding bony structures. While the symptoms reported so often drew attention to the spine, he noted they were 'rarely unattended by irritability, fretfulness, emotional tendency, and inability to confine the attention. These can only be the result of derangement in the higher cerebral centres'. He supported this idea with the following:

'. . . the cerebral centres represent a far higher development of function, and to perform this function must have a more delicately organised intimate structure than the lower centres of the cord, which preside over the more simple reflex activities of the body. This fact alone should render them more liable to derangement from a jar as resulting from a fall or collision in which both brain and cord must participate.'

The concept of 'concussion of the spine' thus evolved in the later part of the last century from the organic view of Erichsen to the positions of those such as Page and Putnam who recognized that psychological events were of primary importance in the symptom production. The class of injury as a whole it seems could be divided into organic cases, in which clearly observable injuries occurred, and non-organic cases, where injuries were rarely observed and if so were only slight. The non-organic cases were considered further divisible into those called hysteria and others. From the latter group there was a number, not discussed as yet but briefly mentioned by some of the above authors, who were clearly malingering. Walton moved the seat of the disturbance from the spine to the head. These notions clearly represented an advance in the theoretical position, but perhaps in practice things were still very much less clear. A leading article of the *Boston and Medical Surgical Journal* (1883), which had carried several articles on the problem, summed up the position as it was at the time with the following:

'In this iconoclastic age when we are not allowed to believe in a personal devil, or good honest ghosts, or even to coddle our own pet superstitions and hobbies without a suspicion of mental degeneration, it is natural that the medical "bugaboo" raised by Mr. Erichsen some years ago, and christened spinal concussion, should meet with little quarter at the hands of the modern scientific observer. It is possible, however, that in this, as in other things, the sceptic may have gone too far, and that although it was no ghost that has alarmed us there may actually have been some phosphorescent light which we do not understand, and the nature of which we cannot fully explain. . . . A rose, however, under any other name will remain as fragrant to the sufferer, and whether the ailment be termed railway spine or traumatic neurasthenia, the condition is equally distressing.'

References

Boston Medical and Surgical Journal (1883) Leading article, **109**, 400.

Forster, J. (1969) *The Life of Charles Dickens*, Vol. 2. J. M. Dent and Sons, London.

Gowers, W. R. (1884) *The Diagnosis of Diseases of the Spinal Cord*. J. and A. Churchill, London.

Hamilton, A. M. (1906) *Railway and Other Accidents*. Baillière, Tindall & Co., London.

Hodges, R. M. (1881) So-called concussion of the spinal cord. *Boston Medical and Surgical Journal* **104**, 361 and 368.

Le Gros Clark, F. (1870) *Lectures on the Principles of Surgical Diagnosis*. J. and A. Churchill, London.

Page, H. (1885) *Injuries of the Spine and Spinal Cord without apparent Mechanical Lesion*. J. and A. Churchill, London.

Putnam, J. J. (1881) Recent investigations into patients of so-called concussion of the spine. *Boston Medical and Surgical Journal* **109**, 217.

Shaw, A. (1870) In *Holmes' System of Surgery*. 2nd Edition, Vol. 2. J. W. Parker and Sons, London.

Walton, G. L. (1883) Possible cerebral origin of the symptoms usually classified under 'railway spine'. *Boston Medical and Surgical Journal* **109**, 337.

CHAPTER 3

Functional Disorders

In the writings discussed in the first two chapters, the terms 'hysteria' and 'functional' were mentioned on several occasions and their meanings not made very clear. While this was partly on account of the fact that they were to be discussed separately in this chapter, it was also because the users of the words were often imprecise. Thus, for example, Erichsen (1882) wrote:

> 'We will now proceed to the consideration of a condition of the nervous system that occasionally occurs as a result of spinal concussion, which appears in its clinical history, in its symptoms and probably in its pathology, closely allied to anaemia of the cord, and which for want of a better name we are apt to call "hysteria". . . .'

And two pages later: 'The symptoms indicative of this emotional or hysterical condition are. . . .' While he was unclear in his usage of the word hysteria, he nevertheless suggested that the origins of the emotional symptoms were of the same pathology as other symptoms of 'spinal concussion'. Putnam (1881), as mentioned, was far more precise on the matter, and referred to the works of Charcot and his colleagues in Paris. However, Charcot's ideas were not representative of all thinkers on the subject. It is germane to consider therefore, in brief, the origins and ideas surrounding the concepts of hysteria, and their relationship to the problems of 'railway spine', and also to discuss the closely related terms 'functional' and 'psychogenic'.

The term hysteria, as outlined by Veith (1965), had its origins in Egyptian and Greek medicine, being derived from the word 'hystera', meaning uterus. The symptoms of hysteria were thought initially to be related to this organ and its wandering, which having dried up, was supposed to search the body for moisture, and the patient's complaints thus depended on where it came to rest. Several ingenious methods were designed by physicians to entice the errant organ back to its proper anatomical location, including vaginal fumigations. This mode of thinking assumed a unity between physical and psychological symptoms, which continued well into the Middle Ages. The latter however was an era pervaded by devils and demons who were held responsible for patients' maladies, and many people were persecuted as witches who would now be diagnosed as suffering from hysteria or neurosis.

An advance in understanding about hysteria came in the sixteenth century from Edward Jorden (1569–1632). This little-known English physician wrote a book with the grand title:

A BRIEFE DISCOURSE OF A DISEASE CALLED THE SUFFOCATION OF THE MOTHER. WRITTEN UPON OCCASION WHICH HATH BEENE OF LATE TAKEN THEREBY, TO SUSPECT POSSESSION OF AN EVILL SPIRIT, OR SOME SUCH LIKE SUPERNATURAL POWER. WHEREIN IS DECLARED THAT DIVERS STRANGE ACTIONS AND PASSIONS OF THE BODY OF MAN WHICH IN THE COMMON OPINION, ARE IMPUTED TO THE DEVILL, HAVE THEIR TRUE NATURALL CAUSES, AND DO ACCOMPANIE THIS DISEASE.

Not only did this book contain notes on the signs and symptoms of psychiatric disorders but, as the title suggests, also claimed that such disorders were natural, rather than supernatural, and presumably were within the realm of the study of medicine. Jorden, while still persisting in uterine aetiologies, suggested that:

'it is an affect of the mother or wombe wherein the principall parts of the bodie by consent do suffer diversly according to the diversitie of the causes and diseases wherewith the matrix is offended. . . . The principall parts of the body are the seates of the three faculties, which do governe the whole body. The braine of the animall, the hart of the vitall, the liver of the naturall. . . . These parts are affected in this disease, and do suffer in *their functions* as they are diminished, depraved, or abolished, according to the nature and plenty of the humor, and the temperament and situation of the mother.'

He, for the first time thus implied that the brain was involved in the origins of hysteria, and that the brain's *functions* were altered in the disease.

The idea that the brain was affected in hysteria was taken up and elaborated by both Willis and Sydenham. Thomas Willis (1621–73), often called the founder of modern neurology, was one of the great seventeenth century English physicians. He clearly implicated the brain as the seat of hysteria, and explained the situation in the following way (Willis, 1664): '. . . the passions commonly called hysterical, arise most often, from the animal spirits, possessing the beginning of the nerves within the head, and infected with some taint'. He took his ideas further by providing post-mortem evidence to demonstrate that the uterus of patients who had died but suffered hysteria were normal. The animal spirits concept, supported by Willis, was still essentially monistic, and did not invoke, as did his contemporary Sydenham (1624–83) the Cartesian dualism which was later to become the order of the day. Thus Descartes (1596–1650), the seventeenth century philosopher, brought to completion or nearly so, the dualism of mind and matter which was perhaps originally formulated by Plato, and which was cultivated for religious reasons by the Christian theologians. In this scheme, mind and matter were two separate independent worlds. Since mind did not move the body, animal spirits ceased to be the cornerstone of the link between mind and body. As Descartes himself recorded (Descartes, 1649):

'. . . I regard the human body as a machine so built and put together of bone, nerve, muscle, vein, blood and skin, that still, although it had no mind, it would not fail to move in all the same ways as at present, since it does not move by the direction of its will, nor consequently by means of the mind, but only by the arrangement of its organs.'

With regard to the mind he commented:

'I knew then that I was a substance, whose whole essence or nature is, but to think and who to be, hath need of no place, nor depends on any materiall thing. So that this me, to wit, my soul by which I am what I am, is wholly distinct from the body, and more easie to be known than it; . . .'

These ideas permitted the expression of new theories in medical thinking, in that they allowed doctors to postulate natural causes for disease without treading on religious ideology. The influence of Descartes is clear in the writings of Sydenham who observed many cases of hysteria and thought it was prevalent: 'Of all chronic disease hysteria . . . is the commonest . . . few of the maladies of miserable mortality are not imitated by it . . .' (Sydenham, 1740). Hysteria, however, had its origins in the mind: 'The remote or external causes of hysteria are over-ordinate actions of the body, and still oftener over-ordinate commotions of the mind.'

The term 'neurologie' was originally used by Willis (1667) in his book *Pathologiae Cerebri et Nervosi Generis Specimen*, and subsequently became widely used. Robert Whytt (1714–66), the first Scottish 'neurologist', was the first person to define precisely the meaning of the term 'nervous'. For him 'nervous' clearly implied conditions arising from a disordered nervous system, and hysteria was included under the category 'nervous'. He wrote (Whytt, 1768):

'Those disorders may, peculiarly, deserve the name nervous, which, on account of an unusual delicacy, or unnatural state of the nerves, are produced by causes, which in people of a sound constitution, would either have no such effects, or at least in a much less degree.'

It was, however, William Cullen (1710–90), another Scottish physician from Edinburgh, who made the most significant contribution of this era. He was especially interested in the classification of diseases, and his views had a lasting influence on medical thought. He recognized in his taxonomy four principal categories, namely fevers, cachexias, local disorders, and neuroses. The 'neuroses' were further subdivided to include comata, adynamae, spasmi, and vesaniae. The first three sub-categories included such disorders as paralysis and tetanus, and the vesaniae were the disorders of the 'intellectual functions'. He thus used the term 'neuroses' for nervous disorders in general, those which 'depend on a more general affection of the nervous system'. For him these diseases all arose in disturbed brain activity and

'These affections of the mind must be considered as depending upon a certain state of our corporeal part. . . . We cannot doubt that the operations of our intellect always depend upon certain motions taking place in the brain. . . . It is very probable that the state of the intellectual *functions* depends chiefly upon the state and condition of what is termed nervous power. . . .' (Cullen, 1772)

This distinction of the neuroses being dependent on disordered nerve 'motions' was very influential. As time progressed, and knowledge of neurology advanced, many of the conditions described by Cullen became discrete neurological entities, and underlying structural brain pathology identified or at least suggested. However, the neuroses and in particular the disorders he classified under vesaniae, were still associated with disturbed nerve power.

Although other writers around the same time were expressing similar views to those of Cullen, the first use of the word 'functional' in reference to nervous diseases was by another Edinburgh physician in the nineteenth century, Andrew Coombe (1797–1847). It is perhaps no accident that his ideas follow from Whytt and Cullen, since both these men had been at Edinburgh before him.

'Function' as a term had been in use in the English language about 300 years before this, although its use as meaning 'a special kind of activity' had more recent origins (Dallenbach, 1915). There are, from the point of view of this discussion, two main lines of reference. One pertains to a physiological use, that is the activity of an organ, the other to its psychological use, as activity of the intellectual or emotional faculties. In these senses the word does not appear in the writings of, for example Hobbes (1588–1679), Locke (1632–1704), Berkeley (1685–1753), or Hume (1711–1776), in spite of the fact that all wrote extensively on psychology, and Locke had a medical training. Hartley (1705–1757), in his *Observations on Man* (1748) used the word 20 times, mainly in the physiological sense, writing for example about the structure and functions of several organs. Many authors around this time used the word in both senses. Brown (1778–1820), in his *Sketch of a System of the Philosophy of the Human Mind* (1820), however, made specific reference to mental phenomena:

'The innumerable changes, corporeal and mental, we reduce, by generalising, to a few classes; and we speak, in reference to the mind, of its faculties or *functions* of perception, memory, reason. . . .'

Cullen, as noted above, also made reference to 'intellectual functions'.

It was, however, according to Dallenbach, through phrenology that the use of the psychological, as opposed to the physiological sense, of the term became more widespread. Gall (1758–1828) and Spurzheim (1776–1832), lectured widely on such doctrines throughout Europe. While in earlier work, Gall wrote only of 'functions of the brain', later the extended use of the term for psychological reference is clear, and 'function' became synonymous with the older terms such as power or faculty.

Coombe was a supporter of the 'new science of phrenology', which led him to consider the brain and its functions. He said (1831):

'... In prosecuting our researches into what are erroneously called mental diseases, we must ... study the nature of the organic disorder which disturbs *mental functions*.'

However, he then reverted to the physiological use of the term:

'In accordance with the view we have elsewhere taken the exciting causes may be divided into the two great classes of local and *functional*.'

He continued:

'The *functional causes*, then, which have a reference to the brain as the seat of feeling and thought, are not only the most frequent and most important, but in the strictest sense *functional*. ... The term *functional* has a reference to disorder in the action of the organs of mind. ...'

The psychological meaning of the term functional continued in use alongside the physiological, both often being used in the same text. Some neurologists, however, following the lead of Coombe, split neurological illness into 'organic' and 'functional' categories, using the latter in its physiological sense.

The ideas of Reynolds and Gowers provide examples of such thinking. Reynolds (1828–96), writing on the symptoms of disease said that they 'resolve themselves into modifications of structure such as hypertrophy, variolous pustules, etc., and of *function*, as for example paralysis, convulsions, flux and the like'. He took up the challenge of some contemporary authors that functional disease did not exist, by pointing out that there was an obvious relation between functional and structural disease. Thus 'the immediate conditions of all such symptoms as result from modified functions being the intimate organic (vegetal) processes of the tissues ... the mechanical changes ... do not cause the symptoms directly, but by the intervention of secondary induced alterations in the minute organic processes' (Reynolds, 1855). The two were thus mutually interdependent and related.

Gowers (1893) in his well-known textbook *A Manual of Diseases of the Nervous System* divided neurological disorders into organic and functional disease. The latter included 'those diseases that consist only in a disturbance of *function* . . . and many diseases which have this in common with true *functional* disease, that they are transient and not permanent, and that they are not known to depend on organic changes'. He went on to say:

'Molecular changes in nutrition, considered as such, must be colossal to be detected. Such alterations, not sufficient to be seen, but still considerable, probably constitute the morbid process in many diseases that are commonly classed as *"functional"*.'

In his text, under the heading 'functional' are included such disorders as chorea, paralysis agitans, tetanus, epilepsy, and migraine. They keep company with hysteria, of which Gowers said:

'The primary derangement is in the higher cerebral centres, but the functions of the lower centres in the brain, of the spinal cord, and of the sympathetic system, may be secondarily disordered.'

Hughlings Jackson (1835–1911) (Taylor 1958) also considered the use of the term functional. He said:

'it is sometimes used as a name for minute changes, or for those the existence of which we are obliged to discover post-mortem. For instance, it is said that epilepsy and chorea are functional diseases, it being meant that the changes on which the symptoms depend are so slight that they do not involve alteration of structure, but only of function. . . . I have . . . used the term "functional" to describe the morbid alterations of the *normal function* of nerve tissue.'

He went on to consider two fundamental kinds of alteration of function by disease, namely loss of function and over-function. 'In the latter, more nerve force is stored up than in health, and more is therefore expended; the nerve tissue is highly unstable.' He was anxious to point out that functional abnormalities are physiological states, rather than pathological conditions, and that while certain diseases (e.g. tumours) are said to 'cause' convulsions, what really was happening was that the tumour led to neuronal instability.

Of particular relevance to the issue of post-traumatic neurosis are the ideas of the German physician Oppenheim (1858–1919), who originally used the term 'traumatic neuroses'. Oppenheim was a pupil of Westphal, who favoured the view that functional symptoms were due to small myelitic or encephalitic lesions. Oppenheim's *Textbook of Nervous Diseases for Physicians and Students* (1911) was widely known towards the end of the last century. He abandoned the views of Westphal, and attributed the symptoms of concussion to functional disturbances which he assumed 'are produced by molecular changes in the central nervous system' (Oppenheim, 1911). He felt that the term 'railway brain' was more appropriate than 'railway spine', in that the brain rather than the spine was the seat of many of the conditions. Incidentally, he made the very interesting observation not only that any injury can induce post-traumatic neurosis, but that it may also develop after surgical operations—for some reason especially after operations on the ear.

Erichsen, in his book, had not totally ignored the concept of functional illness and discussed briefly hysteria and its role in the production of symptoms. However, he felt that 'hysteria' was a word that 'serves as a cloak to ignorance, and which simply means a group of symptoms all subjective and each one separately common to many morbid states'. He was quite emphatic about its incidence:

'During a hospital practice of thirty years I can scarcely recall to mind a single case in which the emotional or hysterical state . . . has been met with after, or as a consequence of, any of the ordinary accidents of civil life.'

He did suggest nevertheless that it was seen after railway accidents, this he felt being due to the marked difference between such accidents and 'ordinary accidents'.

'The crash and confusion, the uncertainty attendant on the railway collision, the shrieks of the sufferers, possibly the sight of the victims of the catastrophe, produce a mental impression of a far deeper and more vivid character than is occasioned by the more ordinary accidents of civil life.'

Erichsen, however, was confident that making the distinction between hysteria and 'concussion of the spine' was simple. 'It certainly has always appeared extraordinary to me' he wrote 'that so great an error of diagnosis could so easily be made'.

Others, including Page, were not so sure or dogmatic. Paget (1902), invented the name 'neuromimesis' for these disorders, 'because the symptoms thereof are so prone to mimic those which are due to undoubted pathological change'. Page, acknowledging Paget, devoted a whole chapter to 'Functional or Neuromimetic Disorders'. Differing from the views of Erichsen he felt that it was very common to mistake hysteria for structural disease, and that hysteria was a common sequel to railway accidents. Moreover, there was no evidence that functional disorders ever progressed to become cases of organic disease. In one passage Page was again critical of Erichsen. He had just described a case history of a healthy 30 year-old male who developed back pains following a collision, and then had an abnormal gait. The patient received a large compensation award, and three and a half years later was apparently in perfect health.

'That there never was any lesion of the spinal cord the issue of the case has abundantly proved, and we cannot help thinking that such a diagnosis would never have been raised were the influences of the mind upon the body more fully recognised, and were it not unfortunately regarded as almost a matter of course that the injuries received in, and the symptoms seen after, railway collision must be due to "concussion of the spine" and be followed by the chronic meningitis and the myelitis, and the "inflammatory irritation of the membranes" of which we hear so much but which no man has ever seen.'

Page then, unlike Erichsen, clearly felt that nervous shock and hysteria were responsible for many of the symptoms of patients seen following railway accidents. It was a simple step, as already seen, for the classification of the sequelae of accidents to be made logical, by Hodges, into organic and functional. However the term 'functional' was soon to alter radically in meaning. First the works of Charcot must be discussed.

Jean-Martin Charcot, the son of a Paris carriage builder, became Médecin de l'Hospice de la Salpêtrière in 1862, at the age of 37. Of the hospital he wrote:

'This great asylum holds a population of 5,000 persons, among whom are to be counted a large number who have been admitted for life as incurables. . . . We are . . . in possession of a sort of museum of living pathology of which the resources are great.'

He was soon to become one of the most famous neurologists of all time, and by the year of his death in 1893 the framework of modern

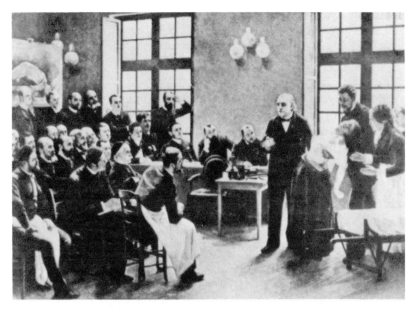

Plate 4 (a) 'A clinical lecture at the Salpêtrière' by A Brouillet. Charcot is seen demonstrating a case of 'grande hystérie'

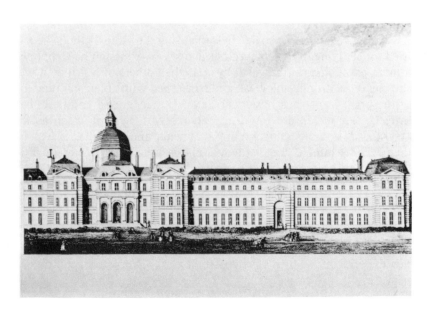

Plate 4 (b) The Salpêtrière

neurology had been laid down. The neuroses were studied at the Salpêtrière between 1862 and 1892, and Charcot was particularly interested in the subject of the post-traumatic neuroses. His work in this field was considered to be great. Pierre Marie said after his death:

'But what dominates the work of Charcot on hysteria, that which will never perish and will continue to serve as a guide to future medical generations, was his demonstration of the existence of hysteria in the male, and his indomitable studies on traumatic hysteria. . . .' (Guillain, 1959)

It is often thought that Charcot was deceived by his patients and that his results were influenced by this, particularly with regard to the work on hysteria. His biographer, Guillain, refutes this. Thus of malingering Charcot himself said (1889):

'It is found in every phase of hysteria and one is surprised at times to admire the ruse, the sagacity and the unyielding tenacity that especially the women, who are under the influence of a severe neurosis, display in order to deceive . . . especially when the victim of the deceit happens to be a physician. . . .'

Charcot began to investigate hysteria using the same methods he had used for studying organic neurological disease. Although he elaborated a more psychological theory of hysteria than others of his time, it was still clearly neurophysiological, and concerned with abnormal function of the brain in various hysterical states. He recognized and described the stigmata which are found in patients with hysteria, such as the anaesthesias and the reduction in visual fields, and attempted to explain them. For example the hemi-anaesthesia 'such as is presented in hysteria—may, in certain cases, be produced by a circumscribed lesion of the cerebral hemispheres' (Charcot, 1877). He acknowledged Briquet's advance in the field of establishing 'beyond dispute that hysteria is governed in the same way as other morbid conditions, by rules and laws which attentive and sufficiently numerous observations always permit us to establish. . . . Thus we are brought to recognize that the principles which govern pathology as a whole are applicable to neuroses . . .'.

He recognized that hysteria affected men as well as women, and suggested it was often found in males after railway accidents. Railway spine and railway brain he felt were in fact manifestations of hysteria.

'These serious and obstinate nervous states which present themselves after collisions of this kind, and which render their victims incapable of working . . . are very often hysteria.' (Charcot, 1889).

He opposed the ideas of Oppenheim and the German school of establishing a separate category of 'traumatic neurosis' for these conditions, and suggested that a common mechanism was responsible for the production of the symptoms in all types of the disorder, whether traumatic or otherwise. He supported his ideas with the experimental induction of symptoms in patients by hypnosis. For example, he would suggest to a patient that when out of the hypnotic state they would become paralyzed after a slap on the back. In that the symptoms he suggested were induced in this way, and were exactly the same as a post-traumatic monoplegia, it seemed as if he had demonstrated the mechanism for the production of symptoms.

Charcot used the term 'functional' in the physiological sense that several others outlined above suggested. Thus in discussing the aetiology of a hysterical upper limb paralysis he said:

'There is without doubt a lesion of the nervous centres, but where is it situated, and what is its nature? It is, I opine, in the grey matter of the cerebral hemisphere on the side opposite the paralysis, and more precisely in the motor zone of the arm. . . . But certainly it is not of the nature of a circumscribed organic lesion of a destructive nature. . . . We have here unquestionably one of those lesions which escape our present means of anatomical investigation, and which, for want of a better term, we designate dynamic or *functional* lesions.' (Charcot, 1889)

Perhaps even more significant than Charcot's work on post-traumatic hysteria was his bringing together of two other key figures in the history of neurology and psychiatry. Sigmund Freud (1856–1939) applied for, and received, from the University of Vienna, a six-month travelling grant, and chose to visit Paris and study under Charcot. There he was introduced to Pierre Janet (1859–1947), and was able to discuss with him the related problems of hypnosis and the unconscious. Later in his life Freud wrote: 'Pierre Janet, Bleuler and others were able to formulate a theory of the neuroses which was scientifically acceptable because of Charcot's concepts.' Both Janet and Freud broadened the notion of hysteria, and with it ideas on the aetiology of the neuroses and in particular the post-traumatic neuroses.

Janet paid great attention to unconscious factors in the formation of hysterical symptoms, and actually used the word 'unconscious' in his writings. He was, however, unable to take the step made by Freud, and still held on to the notion that the brain in hysteria was in some way abnormal and weak. He rejected both a neurological theory, and ideas which suggested symptoms were faked, considering hysteria as a 'psychogenic' disease. There was a basic feature, namely narrowing of the field of consciousness.

'The hysterical personality cannot perceive all the phenomena: it definitely sacrifices some of them. It is a kind of autotomia and the abandoned phenomena develop independently without the subject being aware of them.' (Janet, 1893)

Discussion of the term psychogenic should at this stage be briefly introduced. According to Lewis (1972) it first appeared in the early nineteenth century, and was considered to refer to the 'origin of the mind, or to evolutionary development which had been due to the activity of mind in animals and human beings'. Sommer (1894) introduced it into psychiatry in a discussion on the nature of hysteria, a disorder which he felt was 'evoked by ideas, and influenced by ideas'. It soon established itself to mean 'caused by psychological factors', although various authors, including Janet, discussed the relative contribution of premorbid personality in association with other factors that led to the appearance of symptoms. His theories were not, however, 'psychogenic' in the same sense as those developed by Freud.

In the German literature towards the end of the last century the term psychogenesis was used imprecisely, but the concept flourished with the developing ideas of Freud. While it is not intended to discuss his writings in any detail, his ideas are crucial for the profound influence they have had, not only on the history of ideas generally, but particularly on the development of psychiatry and the split that occurred, in some countries at least, with neurology. Before his time the speciality psychiatry, as an independent speciality from neurology, was not universally recognized. Freud himself numbered neuropathology amongst early specialist interests, and worked with Brucke and Meynert prior to his visit to Paris. After this, however, he devoted the rest of his professional life to psychiatry. He said:

'I abandoned the treatment of organic nervous disease, but that was of little importance. For on the one hand the prospects in the treatment of such disorders were in any case never promising, while on the other hand, in the private practice of a physician working in a large town, the quantity of such patients was nothing compared to the crowds of neurotics, whose number seemed further multiplied by the manner in which they hurried, with their troubles unsolved, from one physician to another.' (Freud, 1946)

He returned to Vienna and was keen to spread the news of Charcot's work and discoveries to his colleagues. In 1886 he presented a paper to the Viennese medical society which has direct bearing on the subject of post-traumatic neurosis. Freud began by telling the members present of his visit to Paris, and of Charcot's concepts of hysteria. He explained the differences between 'grande hystérie' (when special types of convulsions were present), and 'petite hystérie'. He pointed out that hysteria was not due to disease of the genital organs, that it was not malingering, and that it commonly occurred in males. This last point was contentious in that it was still generally considered that hysteria was confined to women. Although, as Veith (1965) points out, Galen ascribed to men a condition resembling hysteria, and this was repeated by several physicians throughout history including Sydenham (1740) (who referred to the male version of hysteria as hypochondriasis, in that the hypochondrium in males behaved similarly to the uterus in females), in Austria, at the time Freud was reporting, hysteria was still considered by many to be a condition of women, and in any case was thought unrelated to post-traumatic illness. Charcot referred to male hysteria both in the 'classical' sense, and also as seen in the post-traumatic cases. Freud presented these ideas and supported his argument by discussing a case of Charcot's whom he had seen in Paris. The patient was a young man who had an industrial accident, and then developed paralysis of an arm. The patient had a range of 'stigmata', and Freud argued that such cases, and also cases of railway spine, should be considered examples of hysteria.

The ensuing discussion on Freud's paper was heated. Ellenberger (1970) suggests that the Viennese physicians were not, however, in conflict over Freud's presentation of a case of male hysteria; several of them attested the condition by commenting on cases of their own, but the main dissent was about his equating post-traumatic neuroses with hysteria.

In 1893 Charcot died in Paris, and with him his ideas and prestige. According to Ellenberger (1970), the good of Charcot, like all great men, was interred with his bones. At the Salpêtrière his legend turned to that of 'the despot scientist whose belief in his own superiority blinded him . . .', and the controversy about traumatic neurosis and male hysteria continued for a few years only. Nevertheless research into the neuroses continued in Vienna. Freud, through his friendship with Josef Breuer, developed further his ideas about neurosis, psychogenesis, and hysteria. Initially working on cathartic hypnosis they found many patients who did not respond to treatment, and altered their methods to develop what was referred to as the 'talking treatment'. Freud became very impressed with the idea of unconscious psychological motivation and went on to develop a complete psychological theory of hysteria. In *Studies in Hysteria*, published jointly with Breuer in 1895, the idea was expressed that the symptoms of hysteria were due to repressed memories of traumatic events, which were emotionally arousing in that they were not permitted expression, and thus symptoms developed in their place. They likened hysteria to post-traumatic neurosis, commenting:

'Our experiences have shown us, however, that the most various symptoms, which are ostensibly spontaneous and, as one might say, idiopathic products of hysteria, are just as strictly related to the precipitating trauma as the phenomena to which we have just alluded and which exhibit the connection quite clearly.'

However, the trauma for them was a psychological, as opposed to a physical event, which was often not immediately apparent, and frequently was defined as an episode in childhood. Sometimes such events were clear, but often the cause was obscured by 'symbolic relations between the precipitating cause and the pathological phenomenon'. Precipitating causes, defined as 'psychical traumas', were 'ideogenic'.

Initially the necessity for some idiosyncrasy in the form of 'abnormal excitations of the nervous system' was invoked to explain the interaction between the person and the trauma such that: '. . . in such people the excitation of the central organ can flow into the sensory nervous apparatuses which are normally accessible only to peripheral stimuli. . . .' Later, as Freud developed his structuralized model of the mind, other factors were introduced, and a mechanism was suggested as follows:

'Accordingly the real traumatic moment is that in which the conflict thrusts itself upon the ego and the latter decides to banish it. Such banishment does not annihilate the opposing presentation but merely crowds it into the unconscious. This process, occurring for the first time, forms a nucleus and point of crystallization for the formation of a new psychic group separated from the ego, around which, in the course of time, everything collects in accord with the opposing presentation.' (Freud, 1920).

Freud himself did not write much on the specific topic of the post-traumatic neuroses following physical accidents, and it was left to his followers to develop ideas on the subject. With Breuer (1895) he commented:

'During the days following a railway accident, for instance, the subject will live through his frightful experiences again both in sleeping and waking, and always with the renewed affect of fright, till at last, after this period of "psychical working-out", or of "incubation", conversion into somatic phenomenon takes place.'

Further ideas are suggested by this short extract from *Psychopathology of Everyday Life* (1914):

'Similarly, to fall, to make a misstep, or to slip need not always be interpreted as an entirely accidental miscarriage of a motor action. The linguistic double meaning of these expressions points to diverse hidden fantasies, which may present themselves through the giving up of bodily equilibrium. I recall a number of lighter nervous ailments in women and girls which made their appearance after falling without injury, and which were conceived as traumatic hysteria as a result of the shock of the fall. At that time I already entertained the impression that these conditions had a different connection, that the fall was already a preparation of the neurosis, and an expression of the same unconscious fantasies of sexual content which may be taken as the moving forces behind the symptoms. Was not this very thing meant in the proverb which says "When a maiden falls, she falls on her back?".'

Otto Fenichel (1898–1946) wrote about the post-traumatic neurosis. In this condition he felt that there was blocking of ego functions associated with regressive phenomena of a variety of kinds. For him trauma that 'upset the entire economy of the mental energy also of necessity upset the equilibrium between the repressed impulses and the repressing forces' (Fenichel, 1946). In addition, the accidents were perceived as a threat of either loss of love or castration anxiety, feelings which until the accident the patient had successfully overcome. Ideas in psychoanalysis altered with time, and the original theories of Freud were modified. One development, which occurred particularly in the United States of America, was that which increasingly emphasised ego function, as opposed to 'repressed impulses' and what may be called the more 'id'-orientated theories of Freud. Examples come from the works of Kamman and Kardiner. Kamman (1951) thus stated that post-traumatic neurosis 'is not an organic lesion but a failure in the victim's total possibilities for adaptation'. The neurosis was 'psychogenic' by which he meant the result of conflicting forces or drives within the personality structure of the individual. The post-traumatic neurosis was seen as a 'reaction', and was in no way related therefore to the type of injury causing it. In compensation neurosis, which he categorized separately from post-traumatic neurosis, although the patient consciously believes he is ill, careful examination reveals a 'volitional factor' with a foreconscious or unconscious desire for gain. The disorder, he felt, was precipitated by environmental factors, one of which was the prospect of compensation, acting in association with personality defects.

Kardiner (1941) undertook research on patients with post-traumatic neurosis that developed during war-time when many cases of neurosis and hysteria which developed on the battlefield were seen by doctors, and their presentation added much fuel to the psychological ideas of aetiology. Kardiner, like some other authors around at this time, concentrated on the ego and its disturbances. Examples of this type of thinking include such statements as:

'There is uniformity in the symptoms of the acute state; this uniformity yields to considerable diversification during the transitional phase; and when chronic, the symptoms tend to fall again into three or four main groups. The one conclusion warranted by this is that in the transitional phase the individual makes many efforts to master the anxiety and in doing so employs every resource found useful to him in his past experience.'

'The traumatic event creates excitations beyond the possibility of mastering and inflicts a severe blow to the total ego organisation. The activities involved in successful adaptation to the external environment become blocked in their usual outlets. . . . The adaptation to the external world is the result of a complicated series of integrations, which owe their existence in part to the narcissistic gratification of success. As a result of the trauma, that portion of the ego which normally helps the individual carry out automatically certain organised . . . *functions* . . . on the basis of innumerable successes in the past, is either destroyed or inhibited.'

Such ideas need not be elaborated further here, but it is important to recognize not only the shift to a psychological use of the term function, but also the advance in thought about psychogenesis which came about by the observations of patients with post-traumatic neurosis in the war situation which represented a fundamentally different approach to psychiatric patients than the earlier Freudian ideas had called for. Symptoms were not now thought of in terms of 'conflict' between two internal systems of the mind (ego and id), but were seen more in terms of a failure of the adaptation of the individual to a new (and changed) environment. 'Adaptation' said Kardiner 'is a series of manoeuvres in response to changes in the external environment, or to changes within the organisation, which counsel some activity in the outer world in order to continue existence, to remain intact or free from harm, and to maintain controlled contact with it.' In this scheme the post-traumatic neuroses were seen as 'the record of the lasting consequences of an abrupt change in the external environment to which the resources of the individual are unequal'. The ego thus fails in its adaptation to the situation and symptoms result.

By this time both the words 'functional' and 'psychogenic' had lost their original meanings. 'Psychogenic', instead of having, as for Freud, some concept of an internal mental mechanism, had become equated mainly with external events, stress, and pressure. As with the early history of 'functional', several authors came to use the term in a non-discriminating way, for example Faergeman (1963) who suggested that 'psychogenic' could mean either 'growing out of innate constitutional factors' or a 'psychopathic condition covered by environmental factors with which the organism cannot cope'. Jorgensen (1956) despaired of the situation stating that '. . . there exists no universally valid definition of the concept 'psychogenesis'. . . . Purely external psychic causes do not exist'. Lewis (1972) quoted several contemporary definitions to demonstrate the current 'shoddy state of the term'. For example: 'Psychogenic disorders of the personality are those that seem to arise largely because of disturbed interpersonal relations, social maladjustments and the like' (Cobb); or 'The psychogenic disorders of man are in fact sociogenic' (Wolf); to the meaningless statement 'Psychogenic, term usually employed of disorders which originate in mental conditions' (Drever). Lewis's own belief was that someone had done a disservice to psychiatry by giving it the term 'psychogenic' and felt it to be '. . . at the mercy of inconsistent theoretical positions touching on the fundamental problems of causality, dualism, and normality. It would do well at this stage to give it a decent burial, along with some of the fruitless controversies whose fire it has stoked'. 'Functional' has been the subject of several manuscripts, likewise ending in disrepute. Gore (1922), a lecturer in neurology at Victoria University of Manchester, wrote a book entitled *Functional Nervous Disorders: Their Classification and Treatment*. After acknowledging the difficulties of defining 'functional diseases' he went on to state:

'Functional nervous disorders are the expressions of abnormally controlled emotional reactions, determined and adjusted by environmental factors and not by any gross or demonstrable pathological lesion.'

Ramsay (1939), in a personal series of injury cases found that 41% developed 'functional (as opposed to organic) disease' in response to the injury. He outlined four main types of disorder: post-concussion syndrome, hysteria, neurasthenia, and anxiety state. The first of these he actually felt 'may be more of an anxiety state', and the seemingly large number of such disorders in his series was a reflection of the fact that in general practice the incidence of 'functional disease' was itself high. The aetiology was explained thus:

'. . . in such cases the soil is ready for the seed; in other words, that some mental conflict or maladjustment to life was already present and that the injury acted as an exciting cause of the psychoneurotic symptoms which developed subsequently. They are usually more prone to suggestion. . . .'

It seems that he was using 'functional' as synonymous with a psychiatric diagnosis.

Nearer to the present, Blake Pritchard, physician to Maida Vale Hospital, while equating functional with hysterical and thus detracting from its broader meaning, discussed the word 'functional', and highlighted why difficulty had arisen with it. He emphasized that both 'functional' and 'hysterical' implied a positive diagnosis. These problems did not present, as is still commonly assumed, as a bizarre mélange of symptoms without uniformity, but had recognizable characteristics, repeated from patient to patient in a similar form. 'If the essential possible characteristics of a functional or hysterical disturbance are absent, judgement should be suspended, further observations made, and further help sought.' He suggested the use of the term functional 'does no more than describe a particular kind of behaviour disturbance, and is applicable when we do not know whether the cause is in the mind or the brain or in both'. He pointed out that the concept of functional disease as due to altered activity of neurones without physical change did not survive the rapid development of neurophysiology that occurred in this century.

'The reason why "functional" did not survive as a precise and useful term was that the notion of function was uncritically equated with that of activity . . . and ceased, on this basis to have any valid significance . . . the activities of nervous structures can be observed and demonstrated: their functions, although they may be inferred and may be asserted, can be neither observed or demonstrated' (Blake Pritchard, 1955)

Contemporary use of the word has floundered completely. Not only does it refer to psychiatric illness generally, but also to 'those conditions in which symptoms and signs result not from any primary physical disease but from conscious or sub-conscious mental processes . . .' (Brain and Walton, 1969). Confusion is such that clinically patients are often diagnosed as 'functional', as if this were an end to the diagnostic process, and it is assumed that by using this term everyone understands, except the patient, what the cause of his symptoms are. The point is well made by this anecdote from Kessel (1979):

'A professor of medicine was consulted by a middle-aged lady with stomachache. On her second visit he looked one by one at her X-rays and then turned to her, beaming, and said: "I'm glad to be able to tell you that they don't show anything wrong." Seeing her crestfallen face he asked her if that was not what she wanted to hear. "Well *my* doctor told me", she explained indignantly, "that I've got a *large functional element.*" '

However, there still exists a line of thought handed down from beyond Charcot, essentially non-Cartesian. That is of a physiological psychology, based on an understanding of disturbed nerve function in 'functional disorders'. Kinnier Wilson (1930), for example, was critical of the clinico-anatomical method, and what he called the 'neurological school of medical thought'. He said:

'Accordingly clinical symptoms are to be considered as

representing either excitation or cessation of function, or a series in which the latter follows the former. Without exception all are *functional* in the sense of being related to function. To attempt to distinguish "functional" from "organic" symptoms is therefore meaningless.'

He followed this with a personal anecdote from his teacher Bastian, who, when told there was a patient on the ward who suffered from functional fits, replied, 'Did you ever see a fit that was not functional?' and said, 'I then secured an insight into semeiology which I trust I have never since failed to maintain'.

Foster Kennedy served as a further stepping stone, and the recent discovery of the neurotransmitters as the final common path. He said:

'In the millions of nerves in the grey matter of the brain and cord, with their enormous aggregation of processes, there exists the complicated mechanism in which are represented our highest mental functions and the mainspring of physical action. In what manner mental processes and emotional states are evolved from or through nervous structure is as yet hidden from us. Our ignorance becomes more plain in those nervous disorders known as "functional", the symptoms of which are subjective. There is evidence, however, and overwhelming evidence, that structural nerve changes underlie subjective clinical manifestations. There must be organic change causing or paralleling our psychic phenomena. But what these may be, the finer strains of gold and silver and the most careful chemical analysis have as yet failed to disclose.' (Kennedy, 1930)

The theme of neurotransmission, and some other current neurobiological concepts of functional disorders will be discussed later. However, the point is made that even though a mainstream of thought developed in the light of writings of Janet and Freud that psychiatric illness and post-traumatic neurosis implied psychological psychiatric disturbance, throughout there has been an undercurrent arguing for a physiologically based psychiatry with all that it implied.

References

Blake Pritchard, E. A. (1955) The functional symptoms of organic disease of the brain. *Lancet* **i,** 363.

Brain, W. R. and Walton, J. N. (1969) *Diseases of the Nervous System.* 7th Edition Oxford University Press, Oxford.

Brown, T. (1820) *Sketch of a system of the philosophy of the human mind.* Edinburgh.

Charcot, J. M. (1877) *Lectures on the Diseases of the Nervous System.* New Sydenham Society, London.

Charcot, J. M. (1889) *Clinical Lectures on Diseases of the Nervous System.* Vol. II. New Sydenham Society, London.

Coombe, A. (1831) *Observations on Mental Derangement: being an application of the principles of phrenology to the elucidation of the causes, symptoms, nature and treatment of insanity.* Anderson, Edinburgh.

Cullen, W. (1772) *Nosology: or a systematic arrangement of diseases by classes, order, genera, and species; with the distinguishing characters of each, and outlines of the systems of Sauvages, Linnaeus, Vogel, Sagar and MacBride.* Creech, Edinburgh.

Dallenbach, K. M. (1915) The history and derivation of the word 'function' as a systematic term in psychology. *Journal of Psychology* **26**, 473.

Descartes, R. (1649) *Philosophical Works.* Trans. and ed. Haldane, E. S. and Ross, G. R. T. Cambridge University Press, Cambridge (1931).

Ellenberger, H. F. (1970) *The Discovery of the Unconscious.* Basic Books, New York.

Erichsen, J. E. (1882) *On Concussion of the Spine: nervous shock and other obscure injuries of the nervous system in their clinical and medico-legal aspects.* Longmans, Green and Co., London.

Faergeman, P. M. (1963) *Psychogenic Psychoses.* Butterworths, London.

Fenichel, O. (1946) *The Psychoanalytic Theory of Neurosis.* Kegan Paul, Trench, London.

Freud, S. (1914) *Psychopathology of Everyday Life.* Trans. Brill, A. A. T. Fisher Unwin, London.

Freud, S. (1920) *Selected Papers on Hysteria.* Nervous and Mental Diseases Monograph Series No 4.

Freud, S. (1946) *An Autobiographical Study.* Trans. Strachey, J. Hogarth Press, London.

Freud, S. and Breuer, J. (1895) *Studies on Hysteria.* Trans. Strachey, J. Hogarth Press (1955), London.

Gore, D. E. (1922) *Functional Nervous Disorders: Their classification and treatment.* John Wright and Sons, Bristol.

Gowers, W. R. (1893) *A Manual of Diseases of the Nervous System.* Reprinted 1970. Hatner Publishing Co., Darien, Conn.

Guillain, G. (1959) *J. M. Charcot. His Life—His Work.* Trans. Bailey, P. Pitman, London.

Hartley, D. (1748) *Observations on man, his fame, his duty and his expectations.* London, J. Johnson.

Janet, P. (1893) *Contribution à l'étude des accidents mentaux chez les hystériques.* Rueff et Cie., Paris.

56

Jorgensen, E. G. (1956) On the concepts psychogenesis and psychosomatics. *Acta Psychiatrica Scandinavica Suppl.* **108**, 135.

Kamman, G. R. (1951) Traumatic neurosis, compensation neurosis or attitude pathosis? *Archives of Neurology and Psychiatry* **65**, 593.

Kardiner, A. (1941) *The Traumatic Neurosis of War.* Psychosomatic Medicine Monograph II–III. Paul B. Hoeber, New York.

Kennedy, F. (1930) Neuroses following accident. *Bulletin of the New York Academy of Medicine* **6**, 1.

Kessel, N. (1979) Reassurance. *Lancet* **i**, 1128.

Lewis, A. (1972) 'Psychogenic': a word and its mutations. *Psychological Medicine* **2**, 209.

Oppenheim, H. (1911) *Textbook of Nervous Diseases for Physicians and Students.* Trans. Bruce, A. T. N. Foulis, London.

Paget, J. (1902) *Selected Essays and Addresses.* Longmans, Green and Co., London.

Putnam, J. J. (1881) Recent investigations into patients of so-called concussion of the spine. *Boston Medical and Surgical Journal* **109**, 217.

Ramsay, J. (1939) Nervous disorder after injury. *British Medical Journal* **2**, 385.

Reynolds, J. R. (1855) *The Diagnosis of Diseases of the Brain, Spinal Cord, Nerves and their Appendages.* J. Churchill, London.

Sommer, R. (1894) *Diagnostik der Geisteskrankheiten* Urban und Schwarzenberg, Wien.

Sydenham, T. (1740) *The Whole Works.* 11th Edition. Pechey, J. Ware & Wellington, London.

Taylor, J. (1958) *Selected Writings of John Hughlings Jackson.* Ed. Taylor, J. Staples Press, London.

Thorne, F. C. (1949) The attitudinal pathosis. *Journal of Clinical Psychology* **5**, 1.

Veith, I. (1965) *Hysteria. The History of a Disease.* University of Chicago Press, Chicago.

Whytt, R. (1768) *Observations on the Nature, Causes and Cure of those Disorders which have been called Nervous, Hypochondriac or Hysteric, to which are prefixed some Remarks on the Sympathy of the Nerves.* Beckett and Du Hondt, Edinburgh.

Willis, T. (1664) *Cerebri Anatome.* J. Flesher, London.

Willis, T. (1667) *Pathologiae cerebri et nervosi generis specimin.* Oxon.

Wilson, S. A. K. (1930) Nervous semeiology with special reference to epilepsy. *British Medical Journal* **2**, 1.

CHAPTER 4

The Central Issue—Malingering

Although the problem of malingering did not evoke much medical comment until the early part of the present century, it must have been on the minds of physicians through the ages when dealing with certain patients. One of the earliest instances of feigned illness was that of Rachel, wife of Jacob. We are informed that in order to hide some stolen goods she put them in the 'camel's furniture and sat upon them . . . and she said . . . Let it not displease my lord that I cannot rise up before thee; for the custom of women is upon me'. In consequence the stolen images were not found (Genesis 32 verse 35).

It is also suggested from the scriptures that King David feigned madness to avoid danger, Solon feigned mania to excite the Athenians and rescue Salamis, and Amnon, son of David 'lay down and made himself sick . . .' in order that he could seduce his brother's sister Tamar when she brought him food for his ailments (II Samuel 13 verse 6).

Galen and Paré both described their thoughts on the subject, and suggested ways of unmasking it (Bassett Jones and Llewellyn, 1917). Instances of malingering were well-known in certain sections of the community especially in prisons and the armed forces. In 1403 it is suggested that the First Earl of Northumberland 'lay craftily sick' to avoid taking part in the Battle of Shrewsbury. The phenomenon was common in the Napoleonic Wars, and the definition of malingering is given in Grove's *Dictionary of the Vulgar Tongue* (1785) as 'A military term for one who under pretence of sickness evades his duty'.

One of the earliest writers to assemble this material together was Gavin (1843), whose book *On Feigned and Factitious Diseases, chiefly of Soldiers and Seamen*, was the outcome of experience in the 'late long wars which devastated France' during which 'a thousand reasons induced the young men to feign disease to avoid conscription'.

Gavin divided feigned illness into four different types: first, feigned or purely factitious, where disease was pretended or simulated; second, exaggerated diseases, where some wasting disease is exaggerated, with or without the patient's concurrence; third, factitious diseases produced entirely by the patient; and fourth, aggravated diseases, which are increased by the patient using artificial means. His own treatise mainly concerned the first group, occurring especially in soldiers, seamen, and those under threat of conscription.

With the advent of the railways and the accidents mentioned in earlier chapters, the phenomenon of malingering for financial gain as opposed to avoidance of danger or duty was clearly recognized. Literature on the subject became extensive around the turn of this century, stimulated by the establishment of various Acts of Parliament relating to employers' liability and workmen's compensation that were passed around that time. Bassett Jones and Llewellyn (1917) demonstrated that the condition was not confined to soldiers. They summarized their thoughts on the problem:

'There is, has been, and always will be, an ambition to gratify, an interest to serve, an advantage to obtain, a duty to avoid, a penalty to escape—in short, a motive for deception.'

Monetary gain they felt was the most frequent cause of malingering. The term 'compensation neurosis' was introduced by Rigler in 1879 after commenting on the increase in invalidism reported following railways accidents with the introduction of compensation laws in Prussia in 1871.

Erichsen dismissed the whole topic of malingering in a few pages, recognizing its occurrence, but suggesting that if care was exercised no-one would be deceived. Page in contrast devoted a whole chapter to it, especially malingering after railway accidents. Unlike Erichsen, who was unclear about the use of the terms functional and hysterical, Page entertained the dilemma:

'. . . it behoves us to remember that exaggeration may not be, nay very often is not, altogether wilful or assumed. Exaggeration is the very essence of many of those emotional or hysterical disorders which are so common in both sexes after the shock of collisions.'

Of the 234 cases he quotes of his own, 32 were cases of fraud or wilful exaggeration.

It is clear that the railway companies were often targets for fraud.

However, the introduction of workmen's compensation in the latter part of the last century and first decade of this gave to a wide group of people the possibility of securing compensation for injury received at work. Thus it became required by the law that employers regulated their business so that injury would not result to others. The Employers' Liability Act, passed in 1880, provided for compensation to 'workmen' who received injury in the course of their employment provided that the injury was not the direct result of negligence on the part of the workman himself. These powers were considerably extended in 1906 by the Workman's Compensation Act. Under this Act, anyone who entered into a contract of service or apprenticeship with an employer was covered, and unlike the provision of the 1880 Act, the defence of 'serious or wilful misconduct' on behalf of the workman was no longer allowed by an employer if the injury resulted in permanent disablement.

In the first six years after the 1906 Act, the actual numbers of accidents in industry rose 44% from 326,701 to 472,408, in spite of the fact that the number of people at work remained the same. Compensation paid in respect of accidents went up in the same period of time from £2,055,370 to £3,361,650—a rise of 63.5%. Over the six years mentioned, the rise was both steady and continuous, and the non-fatal accidents increased at a far greater rate than the fatal. Additionally, the number of slight injuries did not increase. In seeking an explanation for the paradoxical increase in injuries in the moderate category, without similar increases in the severe or very minor ones in the six years following the Act, a Home Office report in 1912 suggested it was directly due to the Act, and that workmen who previously would have continued to work stayed away for the same injuries. A contemporary observer, Collie, who was a physician at the Maida Vale Hospital for Epilepsy and Paralysis, but also a medical examiner to the Sun Insurance Company and other insurance companies, put it even more bluntly:

'Workmen have now a greater tendency to make what they think is the best of an injury which befalls them—that is, get the most money out of it.' (Collie, 1917)

Such scepticism was perhaps justified if it is noted that the Act specifically laid down that an injured workman received compensation for a full two weeks only if he was on the sick list for two weeks. No compensation was paid if he returned to work in the first week, and he received compensation for each day he was off work of the second week. Only if he was on the sick list for 14 days did the compensation date back to the day of the injury. This, for Collie, explained why the number of cases of injury off work under two weeks remained the same, but those for injuries lasting over two weeks rose so dramatically. Taken in conjunction with the figure of 98 % or more of cases settled out of Court, and that from the years 1908 to 1913 the number of cases decided by the Courts in favour of employers rose for the small percentage that actually ended up there, Collie was led to what seems the inevitable conclusion that: 'there are a substantial number of cases of undoubted malingering. . . .'

On the basis of 3667 accident cases examined by himself, he suggested some 8 % were fraudulent. However, he continued:

'the cases in which there is that exaggeration of injuries which is so nearly akin to malingering certainly constitute a most important group for consideration. It is extremely difficult to draw the line between the two classes of cases, and if one did not thoroughly understand the condition of mind into which many people suffering from even trivial injuries drift, one would be tempted to apply the harsher description in a larger number of cases. Fatal cases of accident cannot be exaggerated; in the other category of cases there is ample scope for exaggeration, and I fear the opportunity is frequently seized.'

The suggestion seemed to be that there is a distinction between hysteria and malingering, but that the line of demarcation is not at all clear since it rested upon a certain 'condition of the mind'.

The subtle influences which lead to various 'conditions of the mind' conducive to exaggeration of symptoms are well known and have been commented on by many authors (e.g. Collie, 1917; Miller, 1961). In many cases the unwillingness to return to work is considered important since 'there is in the aggregate, a large number of working-class men and women who, in returning, linger on the threshold of work' (Collie, 1917). Pointing out how susceptible our minds are to suggestion, Collie believed very often that our thoughts 'run along the line of least resistance'. Thus malingering was not necessarily deliberate wickedness, and many people so affected were following self-interest and the path of least resistance, often unconsciously. He continued:

'when dealing with men of the working class who have met with an accident, and who have some other disability . . . it is in a large number of cases impossible to get them to understand that there is no connection between the two, and, therefore, no liability on the part of the employer for *both* conditions . . . There is a class who quite honestly, from lack of mental training, or sheer prejudice, fail to grasp that because one thing follows another the second is not necessarily consequent on the first.'

Collie also pointed out that the longer an injured person is off work, the more difficult it is for him to resume work, because of the loss of routine and the habit. These remarks are especially relevant when the sheer drudgery of what is often called work is considered. Although a small percentage of people do enjoy their work, and achieve considerable satisfaction from it, there are vast numbers of people in extremely repetitive, boring, and dull occupations where little inducement is required for them to alter their life style. This may explain why compensation is claimed so often after injuries at work and not, for example, after injuries at sport; why compensation is usually sought from large, impersonal organizations, rather than small companies; and why claims for compensation are often reported to be more frequent amongst social classes IV and V (Miller, 1961).

Additional factors are also seen to play an important role in the decision to seek compensation. Often, it is not the victim himself who initiates the claim or even suggests it. Spouses, friends, advisers, trade unions, general practitioners, and relatives are frequently the instigators of the process. Cultural factors have also been implicated. Parker (1970) indicated that in Australia, immigrants from eastern and southern Europe were over-represented among litigants in relation to their prevalence in the society and it is apparently popular policy to label them as malingerers. He said:

'Are we justified in calling these people malingerers?. It is tempting to do so when the lump sum settlement is the only thing which cures their unexplained pains and symptoms, and perhaps it fits nicely with our unexpressed feeling that immigrants are inferior specimens anyway.'

He pointed out, however, that it was more a matter of social pathology than individual psychopathology. He quoted Ellard as saying:

'there are a number of things to add together: a need for dependence, a lack of guilt, a culturally-approved disinclination to take resonsibility for one's own actions, an inability to perceive one's illness in accurate terms and a sick role from which status and gain may be derived. Given all these things, is it surprising that if one removes such a person from his culture and isolates him in another one, and then injures him, he should behave in a way which we find hard to understand and evaluate?'

Ellard (1970) pointed out how in southern European, as opposed to Australian families, a sick person is the most important member, and he is expected to maximize his symptoms to gain support from those around him.

Kamman (1951) used the term 'attitude pathosis' to explain one type of psychological position. In compensation neurosis the neurosis was, in part, created by a conviction on the patient's behalf that he had been in an accident for which compensation was available. Resentment, he suggested, could easily follow, especially if there was scepticism on the part of the company doctor or others, and with this went a wish for 'atonement from the privileged' (Kretschmer quoted by Kamman, 1951). In spite of this, he distinguished compensation neurosis from malingering, in that:

'people suffering from a compensation neurosis are just as sincere in their belief that they are sick as are those who have a traumatic neurosis. The volitional intent is at least foreconscious, and it may even be unconscious. However, it is suppressed by fear, indignation and resentment.'

He advocated the Rorschach test, which gave an estimate both of the amount of regression and the 'preponderance' or lack of a true neurotic reaction, as one way of distinguishing between two categories. In addition Kamman proposed a third category termed 'the attitudinal pathoses'. This title was originally used by Thorne (1949), whose ideas were elaborated by Kamman. Essentially the theme was that the resentment was taken one step further with the development of a nuclear core attitude. He said: 'attitudes occur in constellations . . . every constellation has a nucleus of central attitudes . . . one will develop a constellation composed only of attitudes which are consistent with the nuclear core attitude'. Thus after injury at work, no matter how slight, if viewed by the workman in terms of his being treated unfairly, the only attitudes which will be acceptable are those consistent with this basic attitude and ones not consistent will be rejected.

'If he adopts as his nuclear attitude the idea that because he has been hurt he is unable to work, he is going to interpret reality according only to attitudes which are consistent with his basic or core attitude.'

Thus, if the core attitude contains an element that says because he has been injured he is entitled to some special consideration, of which remuneration may or may not be a part, then he will hold his stance against all arguments until the day has been won. However:

'It cannot be said that the injured workman is in this case a malingerer; neither was he suffering from any kind of a neurosis—traumatic or compensation. He and the union were suffering from an attitudinal pathosis which was a global reaction involving not only the original pathological attitude, but also the secondary personality and environmental reactions.'

Kamman thus is giving this condition—the attitudinal pathosis—an intermediate position between compensation neurosis and malingering. It is essentially a form of personality disorder and thus a diagnosable entity.

Good (1942) described the malingerer as a psychopath who had no feelings of guilt about his malingering, but 'although he consciously assumes and exploits symptoms of physical or mental illness, the variety of the symptom adopted (i.e. whether amnesia, gunshot wound, insanity, or paralysis) is, however, apparently determined by an unrecognised masochistic and very infantile dependent attitude. Malingering is a defence mechanism employed by a constitutionally weak ego against a real but unreasonable and intense anxiety'. Here then defence mechanisms, given respectability by Freud and his followers, are invoked to account for otherwise difficult to explain symptoms.

Other classifications of such patients have been adopted, such as Nippe's use of the word teleophrenia (Nippe, 1927) to designate a mid-ground between neurosis and malingering, in which abnormal nervous reactions serve a conscious purpose, or Mock's division into neurotics proper, liars, and mixed types (Mock, 1930). However, one traditional distinction that has been made between hysteria and other disorders, including malingering, is that the symptoms of the former are variable, accompanied by stigmata, and are amenable to the influence of suggestion and hypnosis. Another, which on the surface sounds quite simple, is whether or not the symptoms are developed for conscious gain (see Table 4.1). Huddleston (1932) thus defined malingering as 'the

64

Table 4.1

Condition	Symptoms for gain	Gain conscious
Malingering	Yes	Yes
Hysteria	Yes	No

deliberate feigning, induction, or protraction of illness with the object of personal gain. A neurosis protracts illness, but is deemed not deliberate'. Schilder (1940) suggested malingering was 'the conscious attempt to imitate symptoms to bring either economic or social gains to the individual'. In practice, however, the distinction is clearly very difficult. Not only is the actual form of the symptoms often the same in both malingered and hysterical illness, but there are many people whose knowledge (conscious) of their intentions seems to fluctuate with time. The definition of hysteria given by the 1941 Brain Injuries Committee of the MRC was quoted by Symonds (see Merskey, 1979) as follows: 'A condition in which mental and physical symptoms, not of organic origin, are produced and maintained by motives never fully conscious directed at some real or fancied gain to be derived from such symptoms.' The implication of 'never fully' is that it blurs the simple distinction made above, and Symonds himself seems to have believed that malingering was often to be found in compensation cases, and in all instances of hysterical fugues. Hurst (1940) noted that malingering may result in hysteria: 'a man who pretends to be paralysed for a sufficiently long period may end by genuinely believing he is paralysed.' The opposite phenomenon is also well known and perhaps much commoner, namely that patients volunteer information that they bring on symptoms, but are often unable to state why. Sometimes they can explain events only afterwards, when their symptoms have resolved, but at the time of investigation are seemingly completely unaware of the situation. Further confusion is added by the group of patients who deliberately injure themselves or persistently seek hospitalization and often surgical operations. These include such disorders as Munchausen's syndrome, 'deliberate disability', and polysurgical addiction.

Munchausen's syndrome was first described by Asher (1972), who referred to it as a common syndrome, and defined three types: the acute abdominal type; the haemorrhagic type; and the neurological type. The latter presented with paroxysmal headaches, loss of consciousness, and fits. Bursten (1965) suggested three major features of the syndrome: first, a dramatic presentation of one or more medical complaints with a long history of hospitalization and operations; second, a pseudologia fantastica; and third, the feature of wandering from hospital to hospital. The reasons for patients' behaviour in these cases are poorly understood. Some have suggested drug addiction; the need for board and lodgings; the desire to escape from the police; or even a grudge against doctors and hospitals which is satisfied by frustrating and deceiving. Other suggestions are that the patients' behaviour is related to masochism; a defence against psychotic disintegration; excessive dependency, or hysterical defence mechanisms, although none of these has been convincingly demonstrated. Patients with Munchausen's syndrome are said to be more aware of their manipulations than patients with hysteria, in this sense being similar to the malingerer. However, while 'aware' of what they do, patients are said to be 'unaware' of the actual reasons for why they do such things.

What is clear is that exposure and confrontation in these cases leads to immediate indignation and usually self-discharge, again raising a suspicion of malingering. Psychiatric consultation is nearly always rejected and difficult to achieve, although reports indicate that nearly all patients do have a severe personality disturbance, most appropriately called psychopathic.

This personality disorder distinguishes them from another group of patients, described by Hawkins *et al.* (1956) who presented with 'deliberate disability'. They described 19 cases, 16 of whom were female. The disability did not appear connected to immediate material gain or advantage, but all patients showed skilful simulation of illness, sometimes involving severe disfigurement, pain, or even threat to life. They noted a high proportion were nurses or related to nurses, and suggested that in the production of the patient's symptoms, disturbed parent–child or sib relationships and emotional immaturity were more involved than secondary gain. In particular, evidence of severe personality disorder in their group was lacking. Their noted high rate of medical and paramedical personnel presenting with such problems has also been commented on by others in relation to factitious illness, and identification with physicians and knowledge of medical techniques are probably important features leading to the clinical picture (Merskey, 1979).

The literature on self-damage has been recently reviewed by Merskey (1979). This is often noted in prisoners, sometimes as a response to extreme suffering. Not all cases have a psychopathic personality, and the relationship to malingering is unclear. Merskey concluded that hysterical mechanisms played a part in self-mutilation behaviour. He noted distinctions between deliberate disability and hysteria saying:

'The symptoms or behaviour pattern in deliberate disability or hospital addiction constitute a manipulative form of behaviour which provides a primary emotional gain. In military and prison circumstances there is an environmental gain and perhaps an emotional one as well. Except for the lack of conscious deliberation in hysteria there are thus at best three major similarities between the other syndromes and hysteria, i.e., the occurrence of gain from solution of a conflict, dependency and regression in the personalities involved, and a strongly manipulative effect upon the environment.'

The differences were further exemplified as shown in Table 4.2.

Table 4.2 A comparison of hysteria and deliberate disability

	Hysteria	Deliberate disability
Age	Wide distribution	Majority 15–25
Sex	Mainly female, not to same extent as anorexia nervosa or deliberate disability	Mainly female
Status	Both married and single	Commoner in single women
Personality	Often inadequate, with tendency to dissociation	More effective than hysteria
Intelligence	Broad distribution, but frequently low	Usually average or above
Psychopathology	Symptoms directed to immediate gain	Not usually directed to immediate gain
Suggestibility	Common, often ill-sustained	Rare
Degree of morbidity	Physical suffering or threat to life sometimes present; not common	Gross disfigurement; threat to life common

Adapted from Merskey (1979).

In spite of this bewildering spectrum of presentations of these problems and their overlap with malingering, some authors have laid down firm guidelines for detecting the latter. Hurst (1940) suggested that there were only two conditions that led to the diagnosis of malingering with certainty. One was that occasionally an unskilled malingerer could be detected *flagrante delicto*. Thus, the patient is caught in the act when he thinks he is alone or unseen, or perhaps even is just unthinking. There are many well-known examples of this in the literature. Hamilton (1904) quoted two:

'An instance which I witnessed, and which has since been reported by Godkin, is that an apparently helpless man, who with great difficulty took the witness chair, and after testifying to the absolutely paralysed condition of his right arm, was quietly asked by the defendant's council how high he could raise his hand *before* the accident, and without a moment's hesitation he thrust it high above his head. The same thing occurred in a case against the Forty-second Street and Manhattanville and St. Nicholas Avenue Railroad Company. The plaintiff, who received a verdict of $5,000 for a collection of vague symptoms and alleged injuries and who in the courtroom was the picture of helplessness, made a violent and apparently muscular demonstration of joy when the jury announced her good fortune.'

Collie recommended surprise visits:

'A.U. detained me a suspiciously long time at his front door. Thinking that he had probably been getting into bed whilst I waited, I ventured to look below the table, which was covered with a table-cloth, and there found his clothes, which he had evidently just taken off. I have no doubt that, had I followed the example of the late Mr. Rose, and put my hands into his boots, I should have found them warm.'

The second certainty for the diagnosis of malingering, suggested by Hurst, occurred only rarely, and that was when a malingerer actually confessed he was shamming. Having given these two diagnostic criteria, Hurst was quick to reassure us that malingering was very rare in the British and the French armies!

Other methods of detecting malingering are far less certain. Huddleston (1932) suggested it was possible to detect malingerers by their attitude:

'The out and out malingerer is usually detectable by various bits of evidence: peculiar attitudes towards the examination—generally suspicious, sometimes sullen, sometimes "smart-alecky"—a certain avoidance of too close scrutiny, often an unusual solicitude for his rights ... generally a mental incapacity to be quite consistent in his complaints. The malingerer shows a tendency to overact his part.'

He felt that one difference between a malingerer and an hysteric was that the former gave every detail of the accident and its sequelae whereas the latter's account contained gaps and inaccuracies. Hysterics are usually cooperative at interview. It was suggested that in the army the simplest way to detect a malingerer was by isolation from his friends, reading matter and tobacco, since in these circumstances malingered symptoms have a tendency to get better.

Bassett Jones and Llewellyn (1917) urged us to look at the eyes:

'It is in and around the eyes that we may discern most clearly the natural language of slyness, cunning, craft or other sparks of deceit. The conscious malingerer is uneasy, fearful of detection, his unrest betraying itself by the restless wavering of the eyes, their sidelong furtive glance through veiled or drooping lids.'

Engel (1970) commented:

'In general, the malingerer is aloof, suspicious, hostile, secretive, unfriendly, and more concerned about his symptoms; the patient with conversion is more dependant, appealing, clinging, and although clearly acting out the sick role, shows less than the expected concern about the symptom. ... Amelioration of symptoms with the establishment of an effective relationship with the physician is more characteristic of conversion than malingering. ... The malingerer may be reluctant to co-operate in diagnostic procedures which unmask him; the conversion patient is eager for confirmation of an organic explanation for his symptoms.'

Time is often held to be important, in that with prolonged examinations the malingerer is more likely to give his game away, thus fulfilling one of Hurst's criteria.

It is then clear that while theoretically the distinction between malingering and hysteria is thought to reside in the differentiation between conscious and unconscious mechanisms, in reality the

distinction is very difficult, and several authors have added more
confusion by invoking unconscious mechanisms in malingering.
Others are highly critical, if not hostile, to this differentiation. Rosanoff
(1929) felt that traumatic hysteria and malingering were essentially the
same, for they were both motivated by a desire for compensation.
Miller (1961) was not alone, but perhaps was one of the more
outspoken of the antagonists. Thus he said:

'Many of those intimately concerned with compensation work—
and here I refer to trade union and insurance officers as well as to
judges, barristers and solicitors—are convinced that it
(malingering) is far from uncommon in these cases, and deplore
the inability of doctors to recognise the condition or their
hesitancy in expressing an opinion in this connection to which
they will freely admit in private conversation.'

On the distinction between conscious and unconscious motives, he is
clear that:

'differentiation . . . is quite insusceptible to any form of scientific
inquiry, and it depends on nothing more infallible than one man's
assessment of what is probably going on in another man's
mind. . . . Whether exaggeration and simulation are "conscious"
or "unconscious" their only purpose is to make the observer
believe that the disability is greater than it really is. To compensate
a man financially because he is stated to be deceiving himself as
well as trying to deceive others is strange equity and stranger
logic.'

Miller's conclusions were based on one review of 47 of 200
consecutive cases of head injury who had psychoneurotic symptoms.
He found that such complaints were twice as common with industrial
as opposed to road traffic accidents, especially if the employers were
large industrial organizations or nationalized industries; that it was
twice as common in men as opposed to women (whereas neurosis
generally is considered to occur more frequently in women); that there
was an inverse relationship between the neurosis and the severity of the
injury and the duration of the unconsciousness; and that it was more
prevalent in patients in the social class groups IV and V. He described
the behaviour of a typical patient, which merits inclusion in full:

'The behaviour of the patient with accident neurosis at the

consultation is characteristic. If he is being examined at the request of the insurance company he frequently arrives late. He is invariably accompanied, often by a member of his family, who does not wait to be invited into the consulting room, but who resolutely enters with him, and more often than not takes an active part in the consultation, speaking for him, prompting him, and reminding him of symptoms that may for the moment have slipped his memory. The patient's attitude is one of martyred gloom, but he is also very much on the defensive, and exudes hostility, especially at any suggestion that his condition may be improving. It is almost impossible to conjure up a smile to relax his appearance of preoccupied tension. His complaint of amnesia is often at variance with the circumstantial detail which invests his account of the events that led up to the accident many months ago. At some stage he will often insist that the cause of this was absolutely outside his control and that it was entirely due to someone else's fault. The "someone else" is rarely specified, but is usually "they"—in some vague way identified with the employing organisation—or the unknown other motorist.

'The most consistent clinical feature is the subject's unshakable conviction of unfitness for work, a conviction quite unrelated to overt disability even if his symptomatology is accepted at its face value. At a later stage the patient will declare his fitness for light work, which is not often available. The logic of prescribing light duties rather than his customary employment for the rehabilitation of the neurotic worker may appear obscure, but the reason why such a recommendation is often made by the general practitioner and echoed in consultant reports is clear: light work is better than no work at all, and it is generally appreciated that unless the doctor goes halfway to meet him—and especially if he provokes actual hostility—the patient's complaints will be intensified and disability further prolonged. The equanimity with which these patients will accept the tedium of months or even years of idleness, apparently unmitigated by any pleasurable diversion, is remarkable.

'Another cardinal feature is an absolute refusal to admit any degree of symptomatic improvement. With the exception of a few well-defined conditions such as traumatic arthritis and causalgia, there are no physical results of injury the discomforts of which do not in the course of time become somewhat less intense. Far from accepting the suggestion of such improvement these patients often make the improbable claim that pain at the site of injury has steadily become more severe over a period of months or years.'

Miller's view of post-traumatic neurosis was that it was essentially the outcome of the setting in which it occurred. It was related to a 'lack of social responsibility'. The hypothetical response of the injured workman who has just come round after a brick has fallen on his head was not 'Where am I?' but 'Whose brick was it?'

'He discusses the incident with his friends, and consults a Union official, who encourages him to formulate a claim . . . his doctor acquiesces in his suggestion of a week's rest.'

A process has been initiated and there follows a period when the patient sees little of his doctor but has a great number of consultations with solicitors, union officials and medical consultants.

'With repeated examinations and interrogations the familiar syndrome assumes its usual florid form.'

Miller supported these ideas with his own follow-up studies. He pointed out that few such studies of patients after settlement had been described, and these were inadequate. He presents data on 50 of his patients. All had disabling nervous symptoms, 31 after industrial and 18 after road traffic accidents. Only two of these were disabled by their symptoms at re-examination two years after their claim had been settled and recovery in 45 of the patients had been complete. At follow-up both contractures and occupational phobias cleared, and the majority of patients with the so-called predisposition to neurosis recovered and lost their symptoms. Miller concluded:

'. . . it is not the result of the accident but a concomitant of the compensation and a manifestation of the hope of financial gain. . . . Accident neurosis is not an entirely homogenous syndrome, but presents a spectrum ranging from gross conversion hysteria at the end of the scale to frank malingering at the other. To accept these cases uncritically as instances of hysteria is to concede a general unconsciousness of motivation which strains my credulity. Indeed, what "evidence" is available on this issue points rather in the opposite direction.'

In reality, hardly any experimental work has been carried out on malingering. The brief literature on simulation of mental illness was reviewed by Anderson *et al.* (1959), who reported their own investigations on 18 students who were asked to mimic mental disorder. The subjects were asked to imagine they had committed murder, and were to feign madness to escape the consequences. Three groups of controls were also examined; a normal group of volunteers, a group of patients with organic dementia, and a group with the Ganser syndrome of pseudodementia. None of the experimental group was able to produce a pattern that closely resembled any well-defined psychiatric illness, although the commonest attempted was depression. The authors found that the length and thoroughness of the examination was important for revealing simulation, and with fatigue the experimental group's responses became more and more normal.

No account of malingering would be worthwhile without brief mention of the writings of Richard Asher. Although not specifically discussing post-traumatic neurosis he had some interesting and amusing things to say about the subject (Asher, 1972). He defined malingering as 'the imitation, production or encouragement of illness for a deliberate end' and, as others, suggested the patient is quite conscious of what he is doing and why he is doing it. Hysterics he felt were unaware of what they were doing. As defined, malingering was a rare condition. He classified malingering into three types dependent on motive: fear, desire, and escape. Compensation clearly fell into the second category whereas malingering in the forces would be in the first group. With a sense of caution about the whole concept he wrote:

'The pride of a doctor who has caught a malingerer is alike to that of a fisherman who has landed an enormous fish and his stories (like those of fishermen) may become somewhat exaggerated in the telling.'

References

Anderson, E. W., Trethowan, W. H. and Kenna, J. C. (1959) An experimental investigation of simulation and pseudodementia. *Acta Psychiatrica et Neurologica Scandinavica* **34**, Suppl. 132.

Asher, R. (1972) *Talking Sense—a Selection of his Papers.* Ed. Sir Francis Avery Jones. Pitman Medical Publishing, London.

Bassett Jones, A. and Llewellyn, L. J. (1917) *Malingering or the Simulation of Disease.* William Heinemann, London.

Bursten, B. (1965) On Munchausen's syndrome. *Archives of General Psychiatry* **13**, 261.

Collie, J. (1917) *Malingering and Feigned Sickness.* Edward Arnold, London.

Ellard, J. (1970) Psychological reactions to compensable injury. *Medical Journal of Australia* **2**, 349.

Engel, G. L. (1970) Conversion symptoms. In *Signs and Symptoms*. 5th Edition, p. 650. Ed. MacBryde, C. M. and Blacklow, R. S. Lippincott, Philadelphia.

Gavin, H. (1843) *On Feigned and Factitious Diseases Chiefly of Soldiers and Seamen*. J. Churchill, London.

Good, R. (1942) Malingering. *British Medical Journal* **2**, 359.

Hamilton, A. M. (1904) *Railway and Other Accidents*. Baillière Tindall and Co, London.

Hawkins, J. R., Jones, K. S., Sim, M. and Tibbetts, R. W. (1956) Deliberate Disability. *British Medical Journal* **1**, 361.

Huddleston, J. H. (1932) *Accidents, Neuroses and Compensation*. Williams and Wilkins, Baltimore.

Hurst, A. F. (1940) *Medical Diseases of War*. Edward Arnold, London.

Kamman, G. R. (1951) Traumatic neurosis, compensation neurosis or attitude pathosis? *Archives of Neurology and Psychiatry* **65**, 593.

Merskey, H. (1979) *The Analysis of Hysteria*. Baillière Tindall, London.

Miller, H. (1961) Accident Neuroses. *British Medical Journal* **1**, 919.

Mock, H. E. (1930) Rehabilitation of the disabled. *Journal of the American Medical Association* **95**, 31.

Nippe, M. (1927) Intentional abnormal psychic reactions. *Journal of the American Medical Association* **88**, 1527.

Parker, N. (1970) Accident neurosis. *Medical Journal of Australia* **2**, 362.

Rigler, C. T. J. (1879) *Über die Folgen der Verletzungen auf Eisenbahnen*. Reimer, Berlin.

Rosanoff, A. J. (1929) Traumatic hysteria versus malingering. *California State Journal of Medicine* **30**, 197.

Schilder, P. (1940) Neuroses following head and brain injuries. In *Injuries of the Skull, Brain and Spinal Cord*. Ed. Brock, S. Williams and Wilkins, Philadelphia.

Thorne, F. C. (1949) Quoted by Kamman G. R. (1951).

CHAPTER 5

Organic Lesions

Erichsen was not alone in maintaining that symptoms which developed after trauma, especially head injury, in the absence of clear-cut physical signs, had an organic origin. Ambrose Paré (1649) wrote:

'Besides the mentioned kinds of fractures by which the brain also suffers, there is another kind of affect besides Nature, which also attacks it by the violent incursion of a cause in like manner external: they call it the commotion or shaking of the brain, whence symptoms like those of a broken skull ensue. . . .'

Morgagni had also emphasized the importance of a to and fro movement of the brain in the production of symptoms. Early explanations about the precise pathology were associated with the idea of vibration causing rupture of small blood vessels or damage to the brain fibres directly. Gama (1835) wrote that 'fibres as delicate as those of which the organ of the mind is composed are liable to break as a result of violence to the head'.

Throughout the nineteenth century, as pointed out by Courville (1953), the idea that concussion was related to some movement of the brain remained prevalent, and hence the French 'ébranlement', implying a shaking up of the cerebral contents. Others, in contrast, suggested that vasomotor disturbances were the cause, an idea which was later taken up by Erichsen. The major problem of most experimenters, however, was to obtain adequate pathological material on which to test their hypotheses. Page, as has been shown, criticized Erichsen's work on these grounds, but after all Page too had no access to neuropathological findings, and may likewise be criticized. Some neuropathologists attempted to get round this problem using experimental animals. Witkowski produced concussion in animals by hitting their heads against a table. Perhaps not surprisingly after a few blows he induced permanent changes in their behaviour described as 'unsteadiness, weakness and lack of will power' (Strich, 1956). In testing the hypothesis that these changes were the result of mechanical damage, both Schmaus (1890) and Jakob (1913) were able to produce secondary degeneration of nerve fibres above and below the site of injury in the spinal cord of rabbits following blunt injuries. The latter refined this technique, and used a hammer of known weight which he let fall from a known height on to the heads of rabbits and monkeys in order to concuss them. Following a succession of such treatments, when permanent neurological signs had been produced, he did necropsies on the animals that survived and showed degeneration of nerve fibres in the specimens examined. He also observed haemorrhages but felt these were secondary to necrosis of the neurones.

In this century techniques improved considerably, and many experiments have been done to attempt to understand the problem of concussion and its sequelae. Denny-Brown and Russell (1941) delivered blows to the heads of cats and dogs, either by means of a pendulum, or in some experiments 'it was found more convenient to strike the animal on the occipito-parietal region with a hammer with a long wooden handle and head weighing 120 grammes'. Studying various physiological responses with various degrees of intensity of the stunning blow, they were able to reach the conclusion that 'accompanying the stilling or stunning of the lightly anaesthetised animal is a period of paralysis of the mechanisms of the brain-stem . . . it appears reasonable to assume that conscious and intellectual function in man suffers from the same transient paralysis which is demonstrated experimentally in the lower centres'. They were unable to find any evidence that vascular events were responsible for these changes, and could not detect microscopic changes following brief concussion. They commented that:

'The existence of concussion for brief periods with full recovery indicates a reversible change of a degree and of a character not likely to be observed under the microscope. . . . It is concluded that concussion is a generalised reversible "molecular reaction" induced by physical stress. . . . Our investigation does not deny the possibility of intracellular structural change or of severe permanent interference with highly organised nervous mechanisms.

Groat and Simmons (1950), and others, took up this point in a series of experiments on guinea pigs, monkeys, and cats, that were concussed by a single hammer blow. Their early experiments followed on the observations of Denny-Brown and Russell that concussion was eventually characterized by a condition in which the brain-stem centres were somewhat inert to reflex activation, and the ideas of Walker *et al.* (1944) that the physiological basis of concussion was related to depolarization of nerve cells caused by the shaking of the brain, and that widespread central and peripheral excitation then followed as a consequence. Groat and others concussed their animals, during which they measured a variety of physiological parameters and following which they examined the animals' brains at post-mortem. They found in 'experimentally-induced concussion in animals . . . there is marked impairment of excitability of supranuclear motor mechanisms and widespread depression of brain-stem interneuronal systems'. They divided concussion in three phases: basic, early and late. The basic phase was '. . . a fleeting episode in which the brain is overwhelmed by the concussing shock and much of its nervous structure acutely altered in organisation and activity'. All ensuing histological and physiological changes that occurred started in the basic phase, and demonstrable histological changes were observed within a few seconds of a blow. The early phase was one in which damage done in the basic phase was either resolved or, in neurones which were excessively damaged, degeneration occurred leaving, in the late phase, a 'loss of the neural elements which underwent irreparable change in the basic phase, and often . . . an altered functional capacity'. They thus had observed cell lysis and chromatolysis in the absence of vascular damage or haemorrhage. Even following a single concussive blow they were able to demonstrate a considerable loss of neurones in the brain-stem. There was a relationship between the amount of cell loss in some areas, such as the reticular formation and the lateral vestibular nuclei, and the severity of the concussion. They were also able to correlate some of the observed physiological changes with cell loss, such as the failure of the corneal reflex and duration of respiratory arrest. One of their most important conclusions seems to be: 'It is evident that some cell loss will occur in all concussions, even in extremely light ones, and in some sub-concussions. . . .'

As far as observations in humans are concerned, as mentioned above, a major problem was always lack of relevant post-mortem material. However, throughout the literature there have been occasional cases described which supplement the animal work discussed above. These have been summarized by Strich (1956) in a paper in which she described five cases of her own. Thus in 1899

Rosenblath reported the case of a tight-rope walker who fell and was unconscious for eight months. He died, and at post-mortem considerable loss of nerve fibres was remarked on, and this was considered as secondary to the effects of concussion. Strich's cases all had closed head injury followed by dementia. They survived from 142 to 456 days after injury, and their brains were examined at post-mortem. All the brains looked normal to naked eye appearance, apart from some dilation of the lateral and third ventricles. The main finding of interest was 'a diffuse degeneration of the white matter characterised by loss of nerve fibres and the presence of numerous compound granular corpuscles'. In discussing the pathogenesis of these lesions Strich dismissed anoxia, oedema, or vascular disturbances. There was no evidence that any patient had been anoxic; no raised intracranial pressure was observed at any time, and vascular lesions, although present, were clearly distinguished from the other pathological changes reported. She felt that 'the degeneration of white matter is due to physical damage to nerve fibres at the time of injury . . .', although the evidence for this was in fact circumstantial.

Oppenheimer (1968), in a pathological study, also looked at brains after head injury from patients who died shortly after the injury. Using silver impregnation staining techniques, which enabled him to pick out small lesions with a microscope, he found diffuse lesions in a large number of the brains studied. These lesions were of the same nature as described by the earlier work of Strich, but of importance to the problem of post-traumatic neurosis were the results from the brains of five patients who died following trivial cerebral injury consisting of only a short period of concussion. These brains, while looking normal to the naked eye, on microscopy were dotted with microglial lesions indicative of areas of pathology (see Figure 5.1). The point was made that permanent damage, in the form of microscopic destructive lesions, was present after what were seemingly relatively minor head injuries. Oppenheimer also suggested that if injuries were repeated it would be reasonable to expect a progressive increase in damage with further loss of neuronal tissue.

Another approach has been to study the forces involved in head injury. Holbourn, as a physicist, approached the problem differently from his non-physicist medical colleagues. He studied the physical forces that occurred in head injuries, and pointed out that the acceleration forces that were mainly responsible for damage, including the concussion, were rotational rather than linear. Physicians, he felt, approached the problem wrongly but 'the physicist's initial assumption is that damage to the brain is a consequence, direct or indirect of the

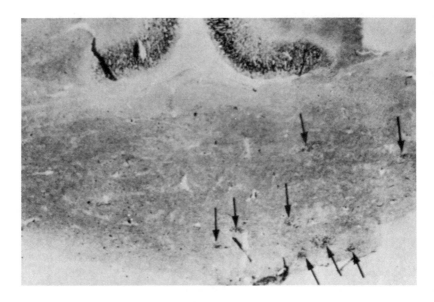

Figure 5.1   Showing microstructural lesions after head injury. (From
Oppenheimer, 1968)

movements, forces and deformations at each point in the brain . . .
these are worked out with strict adherence to Newton's laws of
motion'. Thus forces acting on the brain after injury gave rise to
distortion (shear strain), or decreased pressure, sufficient to cause
cavitation. He backed up this idea with some experiments using gelatin
models of the brain to which he applied rotational forces. He felt that in
the real brain, the non-uniformity of white and grey matter would
cause especially large strains near the junction between them. If the
forces built up in any area of the brain were sufficiently great, then
everything in that region that could be injured would be injured,
including blood vessels and synapses (Holbourn, 1945).

Holbourn's speculations regarding the importance of rotational
movements of the brain was confirmed by the experiments of Pudenz
and Sheldon (1946). They developed a novel technique for observing
the movements of the brain following injury using the 'Lucite'
calvarium, a transparent replacement for the cranium, which provided
a method for direct observation of that organ. While they were not
primarily interested in the question of concussion, and were more
concerned with the concept of focal and contrecoup brain injury, their
observations are important for the understanding of post-traumatic
concussional syndromes. First, they discussed the possible explanations

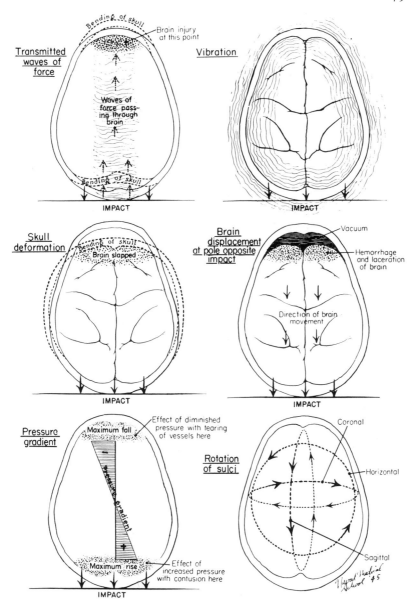

Figure 5.2   Theories concerning the mechanism of coup and contre-coup cerebral damage. The skull deformation shown in the diagram representing the theory of transmitted waves of force has not been described in all of the writings on this theory but is included for the sake of simplicity (from Pudenz and Sheldon, 1946)

for the mechanism of contrecoup injuries under six headings. These were vibrations transmitted from the skull to the underlying brain; wave patterns of force passing through the brain; brain displacement opposite the site of impact; bending of the skull and consequent distortion of the brain; pressure gradients resulting in increased pressure and contusion at the site of impact with diminished pressure and tearing of vessels at the pole opposite the impact; and finally rotation of the cerebral mass within the confines of the skull (see Figure 5.2). Although historically the first of these theories was the oldest, and was supported by Gama, it fell into abeyance in the late nineteenth century, and was replaced by the theories advocating transmission of wave forces. Several ingenious experiments had been conducted to support some of these theories. One experimenter dropped skulls filled with paraffin and coated with ink on the outside, and demonstrated that the surface area covered on impact was greater than that anticipated from the size of the skull, which indicated that a flattening of the skull had occurred. Miles (1892) covered areas of skulls of cadavers with vaseline or glazier's putty, and hit the opposite pole with a wooden mallet. Indentation and coning was observed in the putty, and this suggested bulging. Miles felt that the site of the blow became a 'cone of depression' and at the opposite pole there developed a 'cone of bulging'. At each point momentary vacuums were formed and blood vessels, left unsupported, collapsed and thus damage ensued.

As already noted, Holbourn supported the last of the theories, and suggested the contrecoup could be explained on physical principles in that damage of the brain following injury was due to rotational forces rather than waves of compression or pressure gradients. Essentially these ideas rest on the principle that the brain and the skull move independently but in relation to each other. This was clearly observed and confirmed by Pudenz and Sheldon. They delivered subconcussive blows with a compressed airgun to the heads of Rhesus monkeys fitted with the lucite calvaria, and used high-speed photographic recordings of the events, which were later analysed in slow motion, in order to define the patterns of brain movement. They found that the latter lagged behind the movement of the skull, presumably on account of the inertia of the cerebral mass. The so-called 'convolutional glide', i.e. the amount of movement of brain convolutions, was always greatest in the parietal and occipital lobes, irrespective of the site of the blow (see Figure 5.3). Frontal lobe motion was always minimal, and unfortunately their technique did not permit them to visualize the temporal lobes. They were able to establish not only the importance of the cerebrospinal fluid in dampening the effects of the convolutional

Parietal blow

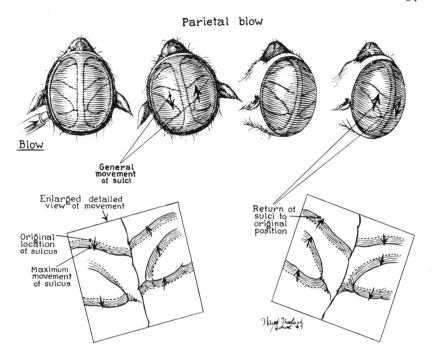

Figure 5.3   Patterns of head and convolutional motion resulting from parietal
blows (from Pudenz and Sheldon, 1946)

glide, but also noted that immobility of the head reduced considerably consequent brain movements. The latter were greater following blows to the temporal and parietal regions, than to frontal and occipital areas. Decreasing oscillations of the brain were clearly visible after injury until the brain came to rest, and such movements were greatest in the parietal lobes where maximum cerebral displacement was located. Associated with the movement of the cerebral mass, they observed stretching and tearing of the surface veins leading to small subdural haematomas.

In discussing these results the authors suggested that their experimental model represented the conditions of head injury in the human situation. They indicated that the lesser motion of the frontal lobes compared with the parietal and occipital lobes is explained by restriction of the former by a rigid anterior fossa, and that this led to strains within the cerebral tissue. Such strains may lead to laceration and softening in the brain at that area and it was probable, although not directly observed by them, that similar strains occurred in the temporal lobes. To support this they quoted the distribution of cerebral lesions in fatal head injuries, where contrecoup damage was generally confined to the undersurface of the frontal and temporal lobes.

These experiments clearly added weight to the hypothesis that head injury, albeit of a minor nature, may cause tissue damage within the brain, the effects of which clinically could be profound. Not only was the mechanism of contrecoup lesions explained, but also the pathogenesis of subdural bleeding which in itself may give rise to brain damage.

Another of Holbourn's speculations, derived from physical predictions, was that some parts of the brain may be more distorted than others, and that 'loss of consciousness might be due to a diffuse neuronal injury . . . to a particular region'. Further experiments in the 1950's confirmed this. Thus Foltz and Schmidt (1956), using Rhesus monkeys, were able to show that following the experimental induction of concussion, sensory evoked potentials, normally recordable from intracerebral electrodes, were absent in the reticular formation, in spite of their continued presence as normal in the medial lemniscus area. The implications of this were that 'since unconsciousness is the single major criterion for cerebral concussion, since loss of sensory activation of the reticular formation results in unconsciousness, and since these two conditions were experimentally produced simultaneously, it is postulated that the unconsciousness produced by cerebral concussion is at least in part the result of the sudden loss of sensory activation, or driving, of the brain-stem reticular formation.'

These results complemented other experimental electroencephalographic investigations which showed abnormalities, often described as flattening, in the post-traumatic period, likened to similar patterns observed after seizures.

Clinical studies too suggest that abnormal electroencephalograms are often recorded in patients after head injury, and generally the degree of abnormality is related to the severity of the cerebral damage as estimated clinically. Jasper and others (1940), in one early series, had some cases of mild head injury that on examination showed many delta waves in the absence of any other neurological signs or symptoms. Although some of these patients were reported as irritable or confused, others were regarded as completely normal. These abnormalities eventually cleared, thus suggesting they were a direct result of the trauma received. Courville (1953), in his study entitled *Commotio Cerebri*, a term once used for concussion, pointed out that one of Jasper's more important observations was that abnormalities of cerebral rhythms were noted to occur in some patients who had not lost consciousness. Reviewing the literature at that time Courville concluded:

'... the impact of a blow responsible for concussion, whether or not accompanied by loss of consciousness, results in a sub-total or complete cessation of cerebral electrical activity, and that this state is followed by the appearance of abnormally slow waves whose persistence is roughly in proportion to the severity of concussion.'

All the evidence of this chapter thus seems to lead to the conclusion that changes of brain function do occur after head injuries, even in the absence of loss of consciousness or clearly defined neurological deficits, and that this is frequently accompanied by neuronal damage and cell loss in selected areas of the brain. Other well-known experimenters, from their own evidence, quote words that would have delighted Erichsen: 'Concussion is the direct result of mechanical violence to cerebral cells. . . . It is a "molecular reaction" induced by physical stress' (Williams and Denny-Brown, 1941; Denny-Brown and Russell, 1941).

Further support for the idea that organic changes occur and are responsible for post-traumatic symptoms comes both from psychologists and clinicians working with post-head injury patients. Reusch (1944) studied the effects of head trauma on intellectual performance by repeated examinations up to three months after an accident. Using selected sub-tests of the Bellevue–Wechsler scale they reported no differences in the degree of impairment noted in patients from a group with fractures and haematomas, compared with a group that only suffered loss of consciousness. However, about half of their subjects showed some intellectual disability. They suggested that most severly affected was 'the ability to keep up a sustained effort, mental speed and visual judgement'. Others have noted impairment of performance on the Halstead–Reitan test battery, on short-term memory and on tactile performance tests following head injury, the impairment being directly related to the duration of the coma. In closed head injury a similar relationship has been found for deficits of non-verbal memory and facial recognition tests. With the latter, even patients with only brief periods of coma or no coma had impairment when compared with a control group (Levin et al., 1977).

Gronwall and Wrightson (1974, 1975) carried out a variety of psychological tests in patients who had suffered minor head injuries.

Their study only examined those with uncomplicated concussion of short duration in an attempt to overcome some of the difficulties of case selection in earlier reports. The main test they used was a Paced Auditory Serial Addition test, which they said gave a measure of 'the rate of information processing'. In this test, digits are randomly presented to a patient, who has to add to the last digit heard the preceeding one (i.e. the second to the first etc.). The speed of presentation of digits can be altered and the percentage correct answers is measured. All their patients had been concussed, but had a post-traumatic amnesia of less than 24 hours and, importantly, none of their subjects demonstrated any history of a previous head injury or any psychiatric illness. They found that patients who showed difficulties with information processing abilities immediately after injury returned to normal on retesting five to six weeks later. Then they selected a group of patients who complained of a typical post-concussional syndrome, and an inability to carry out their normal work. All the patients from this group showed reduced ability to process the required information. As they followed the patients, the post-concussional symptoms receded as the test scores increased. Although their study suggested that a slow recovery in the ability to perform psychological tests was related to a longer post-traumatic amnesia, deficits were seen even in patients with amnesia of less than one hour.

Thus they demonstrated objective changes in intellectual performance that occurred following minor closed head injury, which appeared to improve as symptoms, which are typically those associated with the post-concussional syndrome, receded. They made some important comments about their results. Thus the tests they used seemed to be an index of the rate at which data can be processed. The ability of the mind to deal with information will be inadequate if either there are too many items requiring attention at any one time, or if the rate of cerebral activity is inadequate. Thus for concussed patients, the latter is inadequate and the number of items of information that can be processed at any one time is reduced. The consequences are laid out:

'A patient who has made a good physical recovery after concussion feels well enough to return to work. His intelligence appears to be unaffected, and he will indeed score normally on standard psychometric tests. However, jobs which he could previously have done easily now require simultaneous attention to a number of factors and are quite beyond his capacity, and this he interprets by saying that he cannot concentrate. Stress mounts and with it headache and irritability.'

In a second paper, the same authors describe twenty patients who had a further bout of concussion. They found that the rate of information processing in this group was reduced more compared with those who had been concussed only once, suggesting that the effects of injury are cumulative. This is not incompatible with the suggestions quoted earlier of Oppenheimer regarding the cumulative nature of the neuropathology, and has profound implications for those individuals who suffer repeated head injury, either from accident or as a result of occupational hazards. In particular there is now good neuropathological evidence that the clinical neuropsychiatric disorders to which boxers seem to be prone can be related to brain damage (Corsellis *et al.*, 1973), and a similar situation probably pertains to National Hunt Jockeys, although the actual neuropathology in the cases of encephalopathy described in the latter has not been reported. (Foster *et al.*, 1976). This point was reinforced by the authors, who wrote:

'. . . the most probable explanation of the accumulation of the effects of concussion is that each event destroys neurones, diminishing the reserve available and making the loss evident under the stress of further injury. . . . Whatever the mechanism for this fall-off in intellectual performance, doctors do have a duty to convince the controlling bodies and participants in sports where concussion is frequent that the effects are cumulative and that the acceptance of concussion injury, though gallant, may be very dangerous.'

It is likely that with more sophisticated techniques of testing psychological function abnormalities such as those described by Gronwall and Wrightson will become recognized, as for example in a recent study of facial recognition tests in patients with closed head injury which indicated that deficits were found even after minor injury (Levin *et al.*, 1977).

Various clinicians in their opinions or in the results of their research have supported the above ideas, and come down in favour of an organic aetiology for post-traumatic neurosis. Gowers (1893) for example said of the condition:

'It is necessary to avoid the danger of overestimating the effect of mental influence and of regarding, as entirely due to this, symptoms which are real. . . . The danger is especially great in cases of railway injuries.'

Wechsler (1935) gave an account of 100 unselected cases of head injury seen in his neurological practice, and considered as a separate group those who had no objective signs of brain injury and showed no clear evidence of brain damage. He divided them into four groups: malingering, traumatic hysteria, concussion encephalopathy, and traumatic neuroses. He found only one case of malingering and said 'the rarity of the condition accords more or less with general experience'. The most common sequel of head injury in his series was traumatic hysteria, 75% of the patients having subjective complaints only. This diagnosis was based not only on negative criteria, but also on positive ones, such as an underlying neurotic constitution and secondary gain. He said: 'The accident brings to a head a series of inner and outer complaints which the patient was unable to face squarely or solve adequately.' Echoing the ideas of Charcot he said of the mechanism: 'The trauma precipitates the neurosis, sets in motion the same mental mechanisms as in any other hysteria. . . .' Unlike some physicians who felt that compensation was the most important issue in the production of symptoms, he felt the litigation played only a minor part in the process, and that the trauma was indeed the precipitating factor and in one sense the causative factor of the ensuing symptoms. He justified separation of traumatic hysteria from traumatic neurosis on the grounds that in the latter there were none of the stigmata of hysteria, and the condition affected previously well-adjusted individuals who developed their condition following a life-threatening situation.

In the discussion of Wechsler's paper several authors commented on the organic lesions noted on histological examination in the brains of patients who had been diagnosed as hysteria. Fetterman said:

'Practically all modern writers on the subject are in accord with the author and with Dr Hassin and Winkleman, that an organic basis underlies the emotional symptoms following head injury. . . .'

Attention has also been drawn to the persistent nature and pattern of the symptoms of which patients complain. This had been commented on by earlier authors, but was defined even more clearly by Strauss and Savitsky (1934). They reviewed the literature to the time of writing, and pointed out that the same complaints, such as headaches, dizziness, and fatiguability, occurred in patients who were and were not concerned with litigation. They emphasized that in physicians' accounts of their own head injuries they, 'though before their injuries strong believers in the psychogenic nature of the multiple complaints of patients with head injuries, readily become converted to the theory that these clinical changes are often due to organic disease of the brain'. The authors pointed out that there was a resemblance of complaints in patients of different personality organizations and with dissimilar psychosexual backgrounds.

It was their belief that the symptom complex noted following head injury was an organic disorder due to 'alteration of activity of the intraneural tissues' consequent on the injury.

Courville (1953) examined the post-concussional state and provided some evidence for his conclusion, similar to that of Strauss and Savitsky, that the symptom complex was a clinical entity, as well defined as any clinical syndrome in medicine or surgery. Seventy-four consecutive cases of the post-concussion syndrome were examined. Headaches occurred in 94.4%, psychic symptoms in 79.7%, dizziness in 71.6%, visual disturbances in 52.7%, fatigue in 27%, and tinnitus in 24.2%. The nervous symptoms included anxiety, restlessness, irritability, sleeplessness, forgetfulness, confusion, poor concentration, and sensitivity to noise. Courville, referring to those who believed that these symptoms were all psychic in aetiology, said that the 'neurosis school' was kept alive by some physicians who were employed by insurance companies. He concluded that the same symptoms were found in both adults and children, irrespective of the question of compensation, and that post-concussional symptoms had a basis in structural neuronal damage. He distinguished these, however, from the complaints of post-traumatic neurosis, the main features of the latter being emotional depression, exaggeration of pre-existing personality defects, the elaboration of symptoms both in statement and behaviour, the presence of hysterical components and the multiplicity, changeability, and indefiniteness of the symptoms. The neurosis developed, he felt, in those prone to neurosis, and the traumatic episode with its consequent concussion was the 'exciting episode' in its development.

More recently a group of Swedish workers have examined the psychoneurotic aspects of the post-concussional syndrome (Lidvall *et al.*, 1974). They surveyed all patients who suffered concussion arriving at a hospital emergency room over a two-year period. They followed up the patients, and examined them neurologically and psychiatrically, comparing a group of 38 who had post-concussional symptoms with 45 who did not. Using cluster analysis techniques, they found the post-concussional syndrome was not a unity. While headache and dizziness were the dominant symptoms during the first week of injury, anxiety then appeared as 'the nucleus of the polymorphous late symptom picture'. They reported that a higher percentage of subjects with post-concussional symptoms had spontaneous and/or positional nystagmus on otoneurological testing and that this was related significantly to later reporting of dizziness. However, they diminished the importance of this finding in the discussion of their results saying:

'The absence of associated signs of lesion in the cochlea, brainstem and cerebellum indicates that the lesion in our cases of vestibular dysfunction generally was of a subtle nature.'

There are a number of studies in the literature that have attempted to document in more detail the enduring psychiatric sequelae of head injury. The early work has been reviewed by Stengel (1949). Hillbom (1960) examined data on 415 patients with brain damage acquired between 1939 and 1944, 17% of whom were 'mildly injured'. Of his sample, 30% had either neurotic or psychotic psychiatric disability. Severe neurotic illness was commoner in the mildly injured, although 'anancastic and hysteric' presentations were seen only following the more severe trauma. Similarly, character changes and psychosis were noted more frequently with increasing severity of damage. Generally psychiatric disturbances were commoner after left-sided injuries. In contrast to the psychoses, which were commoner after temporal lobe lesions, and changes of character after frontal lesions, the neuroses were not clearly linked to the lesion site.

Lishman (1968) studied the psychiatric morbidity of 670 patients with penetrating head injury, in whom detailed information was available as to the site and the extent of the brain damage. Both 'depth of penetration' and 'total brain destroyed' were significantly related to psychiatric disability. This finding was not due to accompanying intellectual deficits. He confirmed that the length of the post-traumatic amnesia correlated with the subsequent psychiatric disability and that, if the post-traumatic amnesia was less than one hour, there was an inverse relationship with morbidity. In 345 patients the location of the brain damage was known. He confirmed that left hemisphere lesions were associated with more psychiatric disability than right, and temporal lesions more so than frontal, parietal, or occipital.

In further analysis of 144 patients he related various individual symptoms and syndromes to the site and size of the lesion. Intellectual and behaviour disorders had close association with brain damage, especially of the left hemisphere. While affective disorders or somatic complaints were related to right hemisphere damage, in contrast depression, anxiety, irritability, and difficulty in concentration had only

Table 5.1   Aetiological factors in psychiatric disturbance after head injury

> Mental constitution
> Premorbid personality
> Emotional impact of injury
> Emotional repercussions of injury
> Environmental factors
> Compensation and litigation
> Response to intellectual impairments
> The development of epilepsy
> Amount of brain damage incurred
> Location of brain damage incurred

From Lishman, 1978

a weak association with lesion characteristics. Apathy, euphoria, disinhibition, and the 'frontal lobe syndrome' were strongly associated, and frontal lobe wounds in particular were associated with behaviour disorders. While brain damage itself therefore seemed to play a part in the neuropsychiatric sequelae of head trauma, Lishman (1978) went on to suggest that other factors must also be of importance (see Table 5.1). 'Somatic complaints', such as headache, giddiness, fatigue, and sensitivity to noise, he felt had little clear association with brain injury. He commented:

' "The post-traumatic syndrome" does show some preponderance among right hemisphere wounds and some association with frontal lobe damage, but on further inspection this appeared to be largely due to the presence of irritability as a component symptom.'

From his own studies he calculated that the injury contributed to little more than one-fifteenth part of the total disability, and drew attention to the emotional impact of the trauma which may precipitate psychiatric illness in the predisposed. He commented on the important place that the head held in the body image, and the consequent severe threat that injury to it posed.

Dickmen and Reitan (1977) used the Minnesota Multiphasic Personality Inventory (MMPI) to assess more objectively psychopathology in 27 adult patients consecutively admitted to a neurosurgical ward following head injury, and repeated the assessments at 12 and 18 months post-injury. Significant reduction at follow-up was noted for the scales of hypochondriasis, depression, hysteria, psychasthenia, and schizophrenia, suggesting that the head injured patients complained more of psychiatric symptoms following injuries than would be expected, and that this declined with time. Patients showing significant neuropsychological deficits, as assessed by the Wechsler–Bellevue Intelligence Scale and the Halstead Neuropsychological Test Battery, had greater scores of psychopathology. These findings suggested that the patients with the more serious lesions continued to show neurotic complaints, a result in conflict with some of the other authors, but one which led Dickmen and Reitan to conclude: 'Psychogenic mechanisms are probably overused in explaining the difficulties experienced by head injured patients.'

Levin and Grossman (1978) also used rating scale assessments in 62 patients who suffered closed head injury. The Brief Psychiatric Rating Scale was scored and patients were graded according to the severity of injury. Grade 1, in which patients had only transient loss of consciousness, scored highly on somatic concern and anxiety. Those with severe injuries, and coma exceeding 24 hours, scored highly on several subscores including emotional withdrawal, motor retardation, blunted affect, unusual thought content, and disorientation (see Figure 5.4). Duration of coma was significantly correlated with thinking disturbance and with withdrawal–retardation, but not to hostile–suspiciousness or anxiety–depression.

There are several clinical studies which are specifically relevant to the issue of post-traumatic neurosis. Examination of children following head injuries confirms that a uniformity of behaviour changes are noted, the main ones being irritability, temper outbursts, hyperkinesis, impaired attention, and headache (Black et al., 1969). While there is interplay between the injury, pretraumatic personality, and family setting in the production of these symptoms in children (Harrington and Letemendia, 1958), the absence of compensation issues in this group argues against the symptoms being determined primarily by financial reward.

Taylor (1967) reviewed the evidence for organic change following head injury, and its relationship to post-traumatic symptoms, including the work of Zetterholm that had shown that head injured patients had increased blood/CSF barrier permeability, which was associated with clinical sequelae, and his own work on cerebral circulation times. In the latter, 70 patients with symptoms after injury were examined by using radioactive isotope scanning to assess cerebral blood flow. A reduction of flow was demonstrated, compared with controls, not caused by a decrease in cardiac output, and a relationship was noted

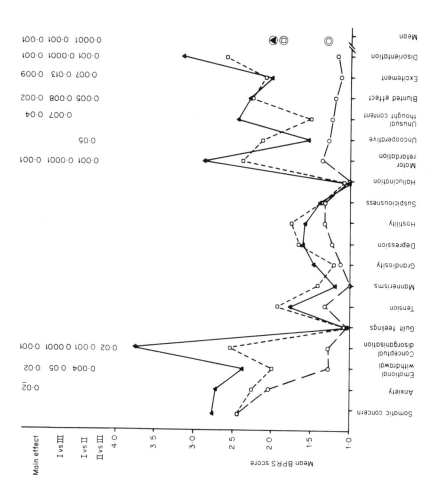

Figure 5.4 Mean score by each grade of injury on individual scales of Brief Psychiatric Rating Scale (BPRS), with grand mean and results of analysis of covariance. Scale scores were adjusted for effects of variation in the injury rating interval. Order of scales corresponds to that of published BPRS. Open circles, grade I; open squares, grade II; solid triangles, grade III. (Grade I—transient or no loss of consciousness; grade II—comatose not more than 24 hours; grade III—coma exceeded 24 hours.) (From Levin and Grossman, 1978)

between improvement in symptoms and the return of the circulation time to normal. He concluded:

'It is no longer good enough to stand firm on clinical convictions that head injured patients, if properly managed, socially adjusted, and carefully rehabilitated, will not have "neurotic" symptoms. The evidence from the few series so managed all points in the other direction. . . . Patients who have minor difficulties in concentration and performance which irritate them and make them act unusually are not "neurotic", they are "cerebrally disorganised" for good organic reasons.'

Several follow-up studies of adult patients have been carried out in addition to that of Miller. Russell (1932) followed up 78 adult cases of head injury in which there was no question of compensation. Symptoms were reported at a lower rate than in Courville's series, but nevertheless occurred in a high percentage of patients. Headaches, for example, were more frequent in those with a less severe injury in terms of the length of unconsciousness. Of nervousness, present in 25 of the cases, and more frequent in those with more severe injuries, he said:

'Abnormal nervousness usually has purely psychological causes and there is no doubt that thinking over a severe accident, especially if foolish relatives enlarge on it, is probably significant to account for the mental state which is so often found. But as the psychological mechanisms which control behaviour are dependent for their smooth working on the intactness of cerebral connections of great complexity, and as these highest association mechanisms are certainly the most vulnerable, it is difficult to exclude the possibility that the symptom has an organic basis.'

Balla and Moraitis (1970) followed up 82 Greek patients in Australia who had suffered neck and back injuries in industrial and traffic accidents, most of whom were reviewed over two years following settlement. The latter had little or no influence on the patient's symptoms, and many with neuromuscular pains were noted to have marked spasm and limitation of movement. Patients with high symptom scores, and in particular those with loss of libido, fared particularly badly, especially with regard to return to work. They also examined the hypothesis that early settlement claims would lead to less morbidity, but were unable to find a significant correlation between this and return to work, as many clinicians seem to predict.

Merskey and Woodforde (1972) have contributed figures, with follow-up of 27 patients who received minor head injury in whom financial compensation was not considered an issue in that any claim lodged had been settled. On reassessment symptoms were still present, and 10 of the series showed little or no improvement. Only two patients were receiving continuing payments, and there was no financial incentive therefore for prolongation of the symptoms. In a later discussion of this issue, where evidence from a variety of sources was taken into account, Merskey (1979) concluded with the following:

'Only in films and television programmes do those who have had blows to the head fall down, stay in coma briefly, wake, shake their heads and proceed symptom-free to rout the villain. Real people suffer longer. . . . My overall experience has been that the great majority of claimants suffer genuine distress, and in Britain at least, recoup from their claim less than they have effectively lost financially.'

In a series of papers, Kelly (1972, 1975, 1981) has provided his own evidence in further support of this view. Miller's 1961 paper, he felt, had been widely read and 'quoted by doctors as an excuse for inactivity and by lawyers in the courts as though it is the general gospel according to St. Henry'. He criticized Miller's own figures, pointing out their selection bias, the retrospective nature of the data collected, and the unfavourable doctor–patient relationships under which they were gathered. Initially, Kelly studied prospectively 152 cases referred with head injuries, and noted between 65 and 75% had neurotic symptoms. Many of these patients returned to work before settlement of their claim, and no relationship was noted between the severity of the head injury and the incidence of neurosis, severe symptoms occurring in nearly 50% of those with severe head injuries. Two-thirds of these patients came from managerial or professional classes, and of 34 patients injured at home or in sports accidents, where no compensation was involved, 24 had persistent neurotic disability. He also attempted a follow-up study of 51 patients who had post-traumatic neurotic symptoms, and were still disabled by the time of settlement. Four had died of non-related illness, but had not returned to work. Of 26 who had not been working on the day of settlement of their claim, 22 had not returned to work, the mean period of follow-up being 2.8 years. In the author's words: 'Failure to have returned to work by the time that settlement has occurred is of bad prognostic significance.' In this series there was no difference in the number of years between accident and settlement in those who returned to work, and those who failed to do this, much at odds with statements often made by others that patients delay returning to work until compensation is settled.

In the light of these findings Kelly's opinion differed sharply from that of Miller:

'In the early days following head injuries there are three organic symptoms, all terrifying to the patient: 1) headache, 2) an inefficiently working brain, and 3) postural vertigo. Added to this is the terror of the accident itself. . . . There follows an anxiety-depressive reaction with the persistence of what were originally organic symptoms. . . .'

His own formulation included the idea that much of these sequelae could be avoided if the problem was correctly identified, and appropriate treatment immediately instituted. In one paper, Kelly (1975) referred to the post-traumatic syndrome as 'an iatrogenic disease'. The majority of patients in his series were told that there was nothing wrong with them, treatment was not offered and no arrangements were made for follow-up. His own contention was that most patients given treatment recover, and return to work before settlement, and the often quoted mythology that the patients only recover after settlement, and that no treatment was worthwhile before settlement, was positively harmful to their future well-being.

Kelly's work is the more interesting since, amongst all the authors who have written on this particular topic, he is one of the few who actually have discussed treatment issues. He acknowledged the benefit of listening, and explaining to patients about their symptoms, and the importance of continuing care after initial consultation or discharge from hospital. Further psychotherapy, psychotropic drugs, and rehabilitation should be planned and instituted where indicated, and return to work needs to be graded, until the patient is able to cope with a full day's work.

In summary therefore, there are many studies that show there is considerable psychiatric morbidity following head injury, some indicating severe symptoms even following closed head injury with little disturbance of consciousness. Neurotic symptoms are not only the prerogative of the mildly injured, and no study has shown them to be clearly influenced by compensation issues. While several authors, such as Lishman, have suggested many other factors which may be involved in the genesis of post-traumatic symptoms, most of the authors in this chapter have cautioned against a ready acceptance of 'psychogenesis' as a cause for post-traumatic neurosis, and there is considerable experimental evidence from animal work to support them.

References

Balla, J. I. and Moraitis, S. (1970) Knights in armour: a follow-up study of injuries after legal settlements. *Medical Journal of Australia* **2**, 344.

Black, P., Jefferies, J. J., Blumer, D., Wellner, A. and Waller, A. E. (1969) The post-traumatic syndrome in children. In *Late Effects of Head Injury*. Ed. Waller, A. E. *et al.* Thomas, Springfield, Ill.

Corsellis, J. A. N., Bruton, C. J. and Freeman-Browne, D. (1973) The aftermath of boxing. *Psychological Medicine* **3**, 270.

Courville, C. B. (1953) *Commotio Cerebri*. San Lucas Press, Los Angeles.

Denny-Brown, D. and Russell, W. R. (1941) Experimental cerebral concussion. *Brain* **64**, 93.

Dickmen, S. and Reitan, R. M. (1977) Emotional sequalae of head injury. *Annals of Neurology* **2**, 492.

Foltz, E. L. and Schmidt, R. P. (1956) The role of the reticular formation in the coma of head injury. *Journal of Neurosurgery* **13**, 145.

Foster, J. B., Leiguarda, R. and Tilley, P. J. B. (1976) Brain damage in National Hunt Jockeys. *Lancet* **i**, 981.

Gama, J. P. (1835) *Traité des plaies de tête et de l'encéphalite*. Paris, Crochard.

Gowers, W. R. (1893) *A Manual of Diseases of the Nervous System*. Reprinted 1970. Hatner Publishing Co., Darien, Conn.

Groat, R. A. and Simmons, J. Q. (1950) Loss of nerve cells in experimental cerebral concussion. *Journal of Neuropathology and Experimental Neurology* **9**, 150.

Gronwall, D. and Wrightson, P. (1974) Delayed recovery of intellectual function after minor head injury. *Lancet* **ii**, 605.

Gronwall, D. and Wrightson, P. (1975) Cumulative effects of concussion. *Lancet* **ii**, 995.

Harrington, J. A. and Letemendia, F. J. (1958) Persistent psychiatric disorders after head injuries in children. *Journal of Mental Science* **104**, 1205.

Hillbom, E. (1960) After-effects of brain injuries. *Acta Psychiatrica et Neurologica Scandinavica*, Suppl. 142.

Holbourn, A. H. S. (1945) The mechanism of brain injuries. *British Medical Bulletin* **3**, 147.

Jacob, A. (1913) Quoted by Strich (*vide infra*).

Jasper, H. H., Kershman, J. and Elvidge, A. (1940) Electroencephalographic studies of head injury. *Archives of Neurology and Psychiatry* **44**, 328.

Kelly, R. (1972) The post-traumatic syndrome. *Pahlevi Medical Journal* **3**, 530.

Kelly, R. (1975) The post-traumatic syndrome: an iatrogenic disease. *Forensic Science* **6**, 17.

Kelly, R. (1981) Paper presented at the Neurological Section of *The Royal Society of Medicine*, 1980 (in press).

Levin, H. S. and Grossman, R. G. (1978) Behavioural sequelae of closed head injury. *Archives of Neurology* **35**, 720.

Levin, H. S., Grossman, R. G. and Kelly, P. K. (1977) Impairment of facial recognition after closed head injuries of varying severity. *Cortex* **13**, 119.

Lidvall, H. F., Linderoth, B. and Norlin, B. (1974) Causes of the post concussional syndrome. *Acta Neurologica Scandinavica* **50**, suppl. 56.

Lishman, W. A. (1968) Brain damage in relation to psychiatric disability after head injury. *British Journal of Psychiatry* **114**, 373.

Lishman, W. A. (1978) *Organic Psychiatry*. Blackwells, London.

Merskey, H. (1979) *The Analysis of Hysteria*. Baillière Tindall, London.

Merskey, H. and Woodforde, J. M. (1972) Psychiatric sequelae of minor head injury. *Brain* **95**, 521.

Miles, A. (1892) On the mechanism of brain injuries. *Brain* **15**, 153.

Oppenheimer, D. R. (1968) Microscopic lesions in the brain following head injury. *Journal of Neurology, Neurosurgery and Psychiatry* **31**, 299.

Paré, A. (1649) Quoted by Courville (*vide supra*).

Pudenz, R. H. and Sheldon, C. H. (1946) The lucite calvarium—a method for direct observation of the brain. *Journal of Neurosurgery* **3**, 487.

Reusch, J. (1944) Intellectual impairment in head injuries. *American Journal of Psychiatry* **100**, 480.

Russell, W. R. (1932) Cerebral involvement in head injury. *Brain* **55**, 549.

Schmaus, H. (1890) Quoted by Strich (*vide infra*).

Stengel, E. (1949) Borderlands of neurology and psychiatry. *Recent Progress in Psychiatry* **11**, 1.

Strauss, I. and Savitsky, N. (1934) Head injury. *Archives of Neurology and Psychiatry* **31**, 893.

Strich, S. J. (1956) Diffuse degeneration of the cerebral white matter in severe dementia following head injury. *Journal of Neurology, Neurosurgery and Psychiatry* **19**, 163.

Taylor, A. R. (1967) Post-concussional sequelae. *British Medical Journal* **3**, 67.

Walker, A. E., Kollross, J. J. and Case, J. J. (1944) The physiological basis of concussion. *Journal of Neurosurgery* **1**, 103.

Wechsler, I. S. (1935) Trauma and the nervous system. *Journal of the American Medical Association* **104**, 519.

Williams, D. and Denny-Brown, D. (1941) Cerebral electrical changes in experimental concussion. *Brain* **64**, 223.

CHAPTER 6

Battle Neurosis and the Question of Predisposition

O, my good lord, why are you thus alone?
For what offence have I this fortnight been
A banish'd woman from my Harry's bed?
Tell me, sweet lord, what is't that takes from thee
Thy stomach, pleasure, and thy golden sleep?
Why dost thou bend thine eyes upon the earth,
And start so often when thou sit'st alone?
Why has thou lost the fresh blood in thy cheeks,
And given my treasures and my rights of thee
To thick-eyed musing and cursed melancholy?
In thy faint slumbers I by thee have watch'd,
And heard thee murmur tales of iron wars;
Speak terms of manage to thy bounding steed;
Cry 'Courage! to the field!' And thou hast talk'd
Of sallies and retires, of trenches, tents,
Of palisadoes, frontiers, parapets,
Of basilisks, of cannon, culverin,
Of prisoners' ransom, and of soldiers slain,
And all the currents of a heady fight.
Thy spirit within thee hath been so at war
And thus hath so bestir'd thee in thy sleep,
That beads of sweat have stood upon thy brow,
Like bubbles in a late-disturbed stream;
And in thy face strange motions have appear'd,
Such as we see when men restrain their breath
On some great sudden hest. O, what portents are these?
Some heavy business hath my lord in hand
And I must know it: else he loves me not.

(Shakespeare: *Henry IV*)

Although since history was first written men have fought wars, and the above quotation suggests that the phenomenon of 'battle neurosis' was known to Shakespeare, the two Great World Wars, and to a lesser extent the American Civil War, were perhaps the most important for furthering our understanding of the post-traumatic neuroses. During the American Civil War, doctors observed the disorder but were at a loss to explain it, relying on a diagnosis which was at the time in fashion, namely neurasthenia, a term originally introduced by Beard (1839–83) to indicate a state of physical and mental exhaustion. Out of this war too arose the observations of Da Costa on the irritable heart syndrome, and descriptions of post-traumatic neurosis, although not titled as such, were to be found in Mitchell, Morehouse and Keen's (1864) work on nerve injuries.

By the time of World War I and even more in World War II, psychiatrists and neurologists were available to observe the syndrome from the viewpoint of their own speciality. Before World War I, post-traumatic problems were considered due to microstructural lesions in the central nervous system, and several monographs on the subject appeared. Mott for example coined the term 'shell-shock' to replace the term post-traumatic neurosis, and felt that the condition essentially was due to a physical lesion of the brain brought about in some way by carbon monoxide or changes in atmospheric pressure (Mott, 1919).

The wars, however, brought to prominence certain observations that raised doubt in the minds of observers as to the aetiology of post-traumatic neurosis. Not only were similar symptoms noted in men not exposed to exploding shells, but also such symptoms were seen to recede when the affected individuals were removed from the danger area of fighting or when various treatments involving 'suggestion' were employed. Southward (1919), in an analysis of 589 case histories of shell-shock and other neuropsychiatric disabilities seen in World War I, noted 'the history of the term "shell-shock" will repeat that of railway spine in the last century: the term will fall into disuse when the cases subsumed thereunder get their exact medical diagnoses—which statistically speaking will prove to be as a rule psychoneuroses, either hysteria, neurasthenia or psychasthenia.' He drew attention to the French distinction between *états commotionnels*, in which physical and chemical changes occur in the brain falling short of producing actual structural changes (lésionnel), and *états émotionnels* when the emotion leads to changes 'after the manner of the normal emotional life, except that the neurones would perhaps deliver an excessive stream of impulses'. For him shell-shock was essentially a psychoneurosis, although he fully acknowledged the coexistence of accompanying neurological disease in some cases.

Myers (1940), who had experience of over two thousand cases of 'shell-shock', divided the problem into 'shell concussion', and 'shell-shock'. The latter gave rise to either hysteria, neurasthenia, or more grave instances of 'mental' disorder, and could occur even in soldiers remote from any exploding missile if they were subject to emotional stress. He thus concluded that the term was ill-chosen, and had generally little to do with shells, carbon monoxide poisoning, atmospheric pressure changes, or problems with 'internal secretions'. He felt 'psychical causes' were involved in the vast majority of cases, which were precipitated by horror and fright.

Neurologists of the day often accepted a psychological approach to both aetiology and treatment of these neuroses, and techniques such as suggestion and hypnosis were widely used. Kardiner was one of the psychiatrists who studied the problem intensively. He observed patients in both World Wars, and developed his thesis along Freudian lines. He collaborated with Spiegel in the production of the book *War Stress and Neurotic Illness* in 1941. He abandoned the system then in use, of classification based on the aetiology of the accident, which had led to such appellations as 'railway spine', or as far as war was concerned 'shell-shock', and stressed that war created one syndrome only, and that this syndrome was essentially no different from the traumatic neuroses of peace-time. Shell-shock, battle neurosis, battle fatigue, and combat exhaustion all meant the same thing, 'they all refer to the common acquired disorder consequent on war stress'. The syndromes seen in World War II were the same as in World War I, although there was a decline in the number of aphasias, paralyses, and epileptiform manifestations. To take their place in World War II fresh cases were 'pervaded by a predominance of affect', with a more amorphous symptomatology.

Ross also studied the problem, and agreed that the war neuroses were the same as those seen at times of peace, the only difference being that in the former some types were far commoner (Ross, 1941). He, in his monograph, divided the war neuroses into acute and chronic patterns. The former were by definition cured quickly, whereas the latter were recalcitrant. However, he felt it was not the trauma which caused the neurosis, and that trauma would not be followed by neurosis unless there was some advantage to be gained.

The concept of gain, so readily apparent in the literature on compensation neurosis, was clearly implicated in post-traumatic neurosis when it arose in such a situation, and was readily detectable.

Thus, observations were made to the effect that post-traumatic neuroses were never seen in prisoners of war, and the speculation was that this was because they had no gain in being sick (Ferenczi and Abraham, 1921). Kral (1951) in a study of patients in an Austrian prison camp, although suggesting that every prisoner at first developed a depressive syndrome, found no new cases of psychoneurosis developing, and said that people with neuroses in prewar times tended to lose their symptoms while interned. Bleuler (1951) stated:

'In the war, therefore, there was not only the prospect of a pension, but also of freedom from the horrors of the front, an enormous amount of material was observed, in whom the severer injuries produced no neurosis, although that alone was sufficient to incapacitate from service and furnish a pension, and that prisoners of war, with few exceptions that could easily be explained, remained free from neuroses.'

The concept, whereby an advantage occurred subsequent to an illness or an accident which led to the prolongation of symptoms, is referred to as 'secondary gain'. Initially, of course, this was seen in purely financial terms, and in the case of 'railway spine' for example, monetary gain was always implied. The concept was considerably expanded over the years, particularly with the advent of psychoanalytical views, to include the realization of suppressed desires for sympathy, attention, revenge, and even masochistic longings. One criterion applied to all cases of secondary gain however—namely, that it shall be unconscious. As discussed elsewhere, if it were conscious and the gain realized, then it would be malingering.

Some authors were sceptical of such ideas, for example Miller's comments about compensating a person for deceiving himself as well as someone else (see page 69). Others, counting such statements as misunderstandings of the situation, felt that the gain, while not actually causing the neurosis, perpetuated it. Kardiner agreed with Ross about the role of secondary gain in the war neuroses:

'The real lesson of World War I and the chronic cases was that this syndrome must be treated immediately to prevent consolidation of the neurosis into its chronic and often intractable forms. The aim was to meet the neurosis before the secondary gain of illness could be exploited by the subject. . . . We know of the secondary gain in the form of compensation for illness after the war. But there is another equally important secondary gain in the form of legitimate escape from duty. The compensation issue then does not in these terms actually create the neurosis but is more a source of resistance in treatment and rehabilitation.'

Kardiner developed his thesis that the traumatic neuroses were a 'type of adaptation in which no complete restitution takes place but in which the individual continues with a reduction of resources or contraction of the ego'. However, the actual character of the neurosis was thought to depend not on gain, but on several factors including the previous personality of the individual, the degree of stress to which he was exposed, his morale and affectivity potential, the extent of incapacity at the time of the initial breakdown and the particular interpretation which the individual gave to his traumatic experience. The last of these factors, in particular the symbolic aspects of the accident, is the one which has received most attention from the more psychoanalytically inclined writers. However, many others have commented on the importance of the previous personality of patients, a problem which will now be discussed.

Babinski and Froment (1918) in their account of hysteria in war disorders gave little space to the subject and merely commented:

'We may remark in passing that predisposition, personal or hereditary antecedents, the nature of the individual and the emotional constitution appear to be of secondary importance.'

Babinski, who had been one of Charcot's pupils, actually developed what he called 'the modern conception of hysteria', which he renamed pithiatism, a word devised from the Greek words meaning 'persuasion' and 'curable'. For him, before the symptoms of hysteria appear they 'require the intervention of a suggested idea'. Thus 'between the emotional shock and the appearance of pithiatic phenomena there is a fairly long interval to which Charcot gave the name of "period of meditation" during which auto-suggestion and hetero-suggestion have plenty of time to intervene'.

In general, however, opinion was contrary to that of Babinski. Both Page and Erichsen had little doubt that some predisposition was involved in those patients who succumbed to illness following accidents. Studying the soldiers who fell ill in World War I, Hurst (1916, 1940) was confident in dividing up the hysterical symptoms into four main groups. These were:

(1) those which were emotional in origin;
(2) those which followed gassing;

(3) those which followed trivial wounds to limbs; and

(4) those which followed injury to the central nervous system.

Each group he said, differed greatly in the 'type of man' involved. Thus, the first was considered to occur in men who were 'constitutionally nervous', and their symptoms were always associated with anxiety symptoms. The third group occurred among 'ordinary soldiers' who never gave a personal or family history of neurosis. The other two groups were intermediate, the majority of the gas sufferers and the minority of the ones with injury to the central nervous system occurring in men of a 'constitutionally neurotic type'.

Kardiner stated his position as follows:

'A commonsense point of view to adopt is that the personality functions which become involved, are those that bear the greatest strain. This really says no more than when a brick falls on a man's head, one does not look for a ruptured stomach. True as this observation may seem, the deep resistance to accepting this as a working basis for evaluating the consequences of war stress is remarkable.'

For him, of course, the personality functions involved in traumatic neurosis were the same as for ordinary neurosis, and they were those functions which helped the individual adapt to the external world.

Lewy (1941), in an article based on his own experience with war neurosis in World War I and traumatic neurosis in the subsequent peace-time, agreed strongly in favour of the predisposition factor. It was clear, he said, that despite warnings from psychiatrists to the contrary, there was little attempt to prevent the drafting of potentially unfit individuals on emotional or characterological grounds. This mistake had enormous financial implications, as well as significance for the future mental health of those drafted and who subsequently developed neurosis. Lewy quoted a figure of 35,846 US veterans from World War I who suffered from neurosis, and each one had cost the American government between $30,000 and $35,000.

Others agreed. Brend (1938) stated: 'Unhurried investigation of war neurosis showed that in all but the mildest cases, there was a pre-existing neurotic temperament.' He supplied figures for Britain showing that the Ministry of Pensions after World War I accepted 60,000 cases of neurosis, 29,000 of which were still on their books in 1938.

Unfortunately most workers expressed their own views and theories but did not produce very reliable data for verification. Some, however, did try to present statistical evidence. Thomas (1943), in a statistical analysis of psychiatric cases, said that there was a history of previous nervous disorder and predisposition in 80% of the war neuroses. Brill and Beebe (1951) collected data on 955 patients of army and navy personnel who, during the war had been treated for psychoneuroses—34% had neurotic traits recorded prior to their service, but 48% of the total were free from emotional difficulties prior to entrance. Stress was the major factor precipitating breakdown. At follow-up 45% had no residual disability, 27% had only slight disability, and 8.3% were recorded as severely disabled. Of the men drawing compensation, the examiners felt that the compensation had no effect in 63% of the cases. Of those still disabled they found a relationship to preservice personality and preservice adjustment—two-thirds of those unfit having symptoms they had prior to service.

Symonds (1943) collected data from airforce personnel. Cases diagnosed as neurosis were analysed, and 79% were found to have anxiety states, 9% depressive states, and 13% hysteria. Two-thirds of the cases had a family or personal history of neurosis, supporting the idea that 'temperamental unfitness for the job was an important causal factor'. They attempted to evaluate the stress involved in terms of length of flying missions and hazard encountered, and found that those with a predisposition to neurosis broke down under mild stress, whereas severe stress seemed required to produce breakdown in men with no predisposition. 'It can be stated that the more flying stress a man has experienced before breaking down, the less evidence of predisposition will be found in his history.' Symonds also collected data on military personnel injured by accidents that were not exclusive to being in the forces, but which may have occurred in civilian life. Of those with evidence of predisposition to mental illness, suspected by either a family or personal history of psychiatric disturbance or alcoholism, invalidism was twice as high as in those without. Further he reported on a group of 111 flying personnel specially selected as being of sound mental constitution by aircrew selection boards. Only 12% of these were made invalid by their head injury, as opposed to 48% for other flying personnel although the injuries received by the two groups were comparable in severity.

Slater (1943), in a study of over 2000 neurotic soldiers, attempted to define more carefully the so-called neurotic constitution. Taking patients referred to a neurosis centre he said of the presenting picture:

'The monotonous character of precipitating cause and clinical picture was mirrored by a monotonous uniformity of the underlying personality. There were few who did not show to some degree a psychic asthenia, a feebleness of will and purpose, coupled with a tendency to worry, pessimism and moodiness or hysterical traits. This was indeed the fundamental disability and indications had been shown in childhood and adult life.'

A family history of psychiatric illness or epilepsy was obtained in 55.7% of the sample; some childhood neurosis was shown by 58.8%; 23.1% had a previous nervous breakdown; and 40% had 'abnormal personality' which was defined as 'a degree of abnormality of personality, in structure and development, which could not be regarded as within the normal limits of variation of the population'. Slater also examined the home environment of the patients with rather inconclusive results. This he felt, was support for the idea that the neurosis was 'a function of bad heredity'. Like Symonds he tried to correlate the strength of the precipitating stress with the symptoms. His results demonstrated that:

'the tendency towards failure and breakdown has to be regarded quantitatively. In some persons though it exists, it is small and needs considerable stress for its manifestation, in others it is stronger, is manifested on slight stress, and is not so readily susceptible to treatment.'

Slater in addition examined patients with organic states, mainly central nervous system disorders, and was able to show not only that injury may predispose to neurosis, but also that in some cases the neurosis would occur with a lesser intensity of constitutional instability.
Slater concluded that the

'two primary re-agents (in neurosis) are the individual constitution and the environmental set-up of the moment. The individual constitution is in the greater part determined by hereditary factors, to a lesser degree by environmental circumstances of the past producing their effects by organic lesions and psychological and physiological conditioning. . . . The momentary environment determines the line of the manifestation, and to a lesser extent the severity and even the form of the symptoms'.

He included 'psychopathic personality' under the rubric of a type of neurotic constitution in which socially obnoxious or partially incapacitating symptoms are exhibited at all times, even when there is no perceptible degree of stress from the environment. Other authors, in different situations, give support to these findings. Adler (1945) studied 200 cases of head injury seen on admission to hospital and followed them up for assessment of mental symptoms. She found not only that 50 % of patients of Latin or Slavic stock developed mental complaints when compared to African and Irish patients (17 % and 21 % respectively), but also that the incidence of post-traumatic mental complications was highest among patients with a family history of psychosis and among those that had pre-existing symptoms of anxiety, hypochondriasis, and depression. Likewise Reusch and Bowman (1945), in a retrospective study of 125 cases of post-traumatic syndromes, found that chronic problems arose in patients who showed a 'much larger incidence of neuropathic traits in childhood: temper tantrums, truancy, delinquency, enuresis, fears, anxiety, obsession, compulsions, stammering or stuttering'. Their study is important in that only three of the cases involved compensation, thus removing a complication of interpretation so prevalent in some of the other reports.

Kozol (1945) classified the personality of 200 patients with mainly closed head injury on admission to hospital, and 43.5 % were assessed as normal. The patients were followed up for at least six months, and those that developed post-traumatic symptoms carefully studied. They found no correlation between the pretraumatic personality and post-traumatic symptoms, the latter developing in 30 % of patients assessed as having normal personality, in 36 % of those with pretraumatic neurotic personality, and in 35 % of those with psychopathic personalities. Noting the slight difference in percentages he commented:

'While the small difference may be significant, it is certainly not sufficiently great to support any theory of post-traumatic neurosis which places chief emphasis on the sole factor of pre-traumatic personality.'

However, he did go on to say that 'in a particular case specific features of the pre-traumatic personality may be the chief factor in the production of symptoms . . . there is little doubt that in many cases it contributes to a greater or lesser degree'.

Lewis (1942) compared the past records of patients admitted to hospital with post-concussional symptoms, with a group admitted with neurosis but no head injury and found no differences, which led him to conclude 'the striking thing is that the longstanding, relatively intractable, post-concussional syndrome is apt to occur in much the same person as develops a psychiatric syndrome in other circumstances without any brain injury at all'. Similar results were reported by Guttman (1946), in a comparison of Forces' personnel with and without head injury who were neurotic. Interestingly both Lewis and Guttman found more people with stable personalities in their head injured groups, although the differences were not of statistical significance.

Hillbom (1960) noted little clear predisposition with regard to depressive reactions but he said:

'In those who react hysterically there has been a somewhat deviating nature—though not always apparent—before the injury. Rather striking is the fact that these have often been persons of somewhat perfectionistic character who have attempted to perform outstandingly, and whose injury has e.g. interrupted a military career of a totally absorbing nature.'

Interestingly Merskey and Trimble (1979), in a clinical study of hysteria in a psychiatric liaison population, noted that while the hysterical personality was associated with an increased incidence of conversion phenomena, those patients with obsessional personalities with similar patterns of illness tended to have organic lesions associated with their presentation.

Dencker (1958) conducted a study using twins who suffered head injury and used the co-twin as a control. The study was not blind, and clinical impressions were used as assessment criteria. He examined 160 twin probands, with 171 head injuries, belonging to 154 different twin pairs, taken from 14,647 consecutive cases with a diagnosis of concussion or a variant of this following closed head injury. Thirty-seven per cent of the twins were monozygotic. Follow-up was carried out on average 10 years after their head injury. The length of the post-traumatic disability was correlated with the severity of the head injury, and symptoms such as headache, vertigo, dizziness, increased sensitivity to noise and light, and impaired memory lasting longer than two months, occurred significantly more in cases of severe injury. However, when comparisons were made between probands and partners a significantly higher concordance was noted for monozygotic as opposed to dizygotic pairs, and he found only a few symptoms that were distinguishing between probands and twins, namely temper, fatiguability, and tension. These he felt were explicable in terms other than the head injury. Factors such as intellectual capacity, rigidity, and viscosity were also greater in the probands, and these were related to the severity of the head injury. He suggested his results led to the conclusion that constitutional factors were more important in the production of post-traumatic neurotic symptoms than the head injury *per se*. Twenty of his probands were said to have undergone a change in personality after injury. However, even before injury, at least 15 had more than their co-twins of the symptoms and traits that dominated the change.

Thompson (1965) compared the pre-existence of neurotic traits in 100 patients with neurological disability secondary to injury, to the incidence in 500 cases of post-traumatic neurosis. Eighty-seven per cent of the latter and 12 % of the former had such traits. He suggested that the accident acted as a trigger for the development of the neurosis in the predisposed.

Lidvall *et al.* (1974) attempted to assess the premorbid neurotic traits of 82 patients who suffered from a head injury, and compared a group who suffered from post-concussional symptoms with the rest. They did not demonstrate significant differences in the variables rated, but their rating scale was 'symptom centred', and would not have included many of the indices used by Slater and others in their definitions of neuroticism. In addition they omitted from their results patients who had reported exactly the same symptoms before injury. When the latter patients were included in the statistical analysis, a significant relationship between the indices of pretraumatic neuroticism and the post-traumatic symptom complex was reported. Using a variety of rating scales to assess psychosocial factors in the two groups of patients they demonstrated poorer adjustment to work three months after the accident, and more mental strain at the time of injury, in the group with symptoms. At the time of the accident, those who developed post-concussional symptoms reported more anxiety associated with the accident, and a fear that the post-traumatic symptoms would be serious.

Recently Keshavan *et al.* (1981) have reported on 60 patients admitted to an emergency unit with head injuries of various grades of severity. Of importance in this study was the assessment at presentation of premorbid neuroticism using rating scales filled in by both patients and a close relative. All cases were followed up at 6 weeks and 3 months after injury and their symptomatology assessed. Eighty per cent had significant complaints at the first follow up and 65 % at the second, headache, sleeplessness, anxiety, giddiness, fatigue, irritability, and intolerance toward noise being the most prominent. While the duration of the post-traumatic amnesia and intellectual deficits most strongly correlated with social dysfunction, the number of symptoms reported correlated only with pre-traumatic neuroticism scores ($r = 0.37$, $p<0.01$). They concluded from these results that physical and social impairments were mainly related to the severity of the head injury, but that subjective symptomatology was related to pre-existing neuroticism.

Many others have also reported that the traumatic neuroses appear with greater frequency, intensity, and intractability in those whose personal or family histories are marked by strongly neurotic trends. As Symonds, generally supporting this view with his own studies, put it: 'It is not only the kind of injury that matters, but the kind of head' (Symonds, 1937). This seems to be supported by the evidence reviewed in this chapter. The fact that much of the work was inspired by the symptoms seen in war-time is not important since several authors report that there is no recognizable difference between the symptoms that develop in the war setting, and those seen in peace-time. In addition the results of peace-time head injury studies lead to similar conclusions. Lishman (1978), after an exhaustive review of the topic of head injury noted the following conclusion with regard to neurotic disability after head injury:

'Clearly these are the areas in which psychogenic factors come into their own, and can often be seen to operate exclusively. Severe neurosis is chiefly found in subjects prone to neurotic reactions generally, and post-traumatic neurotics, when compared to non-organic neurotics, have shown much the same range of complaints and a similar degree of variability as judged by family and personal history.... There is ... a conspicuous lack of relationship between severity of injury and severity of existing neurotic disability, and neurotic symptoms are rare in the presence of marked intellectual or neurological disabilities.... In general it seems fair to conclude ... that the longer neurotic symptoms persist, the less likely are they to be the expression of brain damage.'

A related theme, much discussed but little investigated, is that some people are more liable to have accidents than others. Such patients are said to be 'accident-prone' on account of their physical and psychological make-up. The literature on this subject has been extensively reviewed by Shaw and Sichel (1971) and Whitlock (1971). There are few data available on the previous accident history of people who suffered head injury. In children, Partington (1960) and Klonoff

(1971) were unable to show that those with head injuries had received more previous injuries than controls. However, the accident risk in children has been shown to be associated with both working-class status, and the presence of psychiatric disturbance in mothers, suggesting that the mother's psychiatric illness increases the risk of accidents in their children (Brown and Davidson, 1978). In a study of 100 families with children who were the victims of non-fatal road accidents, compared to a matched control sample, Blackett and Johnston (1959) suggested that accident vulnerability was associated with such characteristics as overcrowding; illness in the family; and maternal preoccupation with, for example, outside work.

The early work of Dunbar (1955) on adults implied that accident-prone people were impulsive, unable to postpone their gratifications, resentful of authority, and had among other features, a history of childhood neurotic traits. She believed that 80–90% of all accidents were related to personality factors that could be identified before the accident. Alexander (1949) suggested that 'accident proneness' was constitutional, and that susceptible individuals could be separated out and excluded from dangerous occupations. Dencker (1958), in his study of head-injured twins, noted that the probands seemed more disposed to head injury than others and concluded 'that accident proneness itself is largely conditioned by constitutional factors, but that the type of injuries sustained is a consequence of environmental factors (e.g. alcoholism) or chance'.

Several studies have tried to assess premorbid personalities of drivers involved in fatal motor-car accidents. Some authors have noted increased psychopathology including depression, paranoia, and increased alcohol abuse, and differences between those involved in single-car, as opposed to multiple-car, accidents. In particular the former are mainly living alone and have higher alcohol consumption. Depressive symptomatology is noted in their histories, and the probable use of car accidents as a means of suicide is obvious (Schmidt et al., 1972).

More recently Sims (1978) has reviewed the literature which indicated that neurosis is associated with an increased mortality. His own studies on follow-up of hospital patients treated for neurosis indicated that the death rate was far greater than expected for a control age- and sex-matched population. While he noted that antisocial personalities may be more prone to alcoholism and accidental death, and that affective disorder is associated with suicide, in the neurotic population there was also an increased risk of death from non-violent causes.

However, the concept of the accident-prone personality as a specific constellation of traits does not stand up to critical review. Attempts to eliminate the 'accident-prone' from various occupations have not proved beneficial, and in at least one study the accident rate for all other workers in an industry actually increased when this was done (Whitlock, 1971). Whitlock (1971) summarized the situation by saying:

'All that one can say is that some individuals have repeated accidents and that numerous factors contribute to these events. The causes of repeated accidents do not remain constant throughout the subject's life, but vary according to time and place and other circumstances.'

There is some evidence that victims of both road accidents and other types of accident are more likely to have experienced change and stress in their lives prior to the accident than others (Selzer *et al.*, 1968; Whitlock *et al.*, 1977). Whether this is related itself to personality characteristics leading to more life events, or to the onset of psychiatric illness is not clear. However, it does seem that current stress and personality variables are interrelated in the aetiology of accidents, and this lends further support for the literature suggesting that in the assessment of post-traumatic illness, pretraumatic personality factors must be taken into account. The consequence for industry, or railway companies, seems clear; the predisposed individual is likely to develop a post-traumatic neurosis. However, the law, as will be discussed later, is often obliged to disregard the neurotic dispositions of claimants when assessing the consequences of injury.

References

Adler, A. (1945) Mental symptoms following head injury. *Archives of Neurology and Psychiatry* **53**, 34.

Alexander, F. (1949) The accident prone individual. *Public Health Reports* **LXIV**, 357.

Babinski, J. and Froment, J. (1918) *Hysteria or Pithiatism*. Ed. Farquhar Buzzard, E. University of London Press, London.

Blackett, E. M and Johnston, A. M. (1959) Social patterns of road accidents to children. *British Medical Journal* **1**, 409.

Bleuler, E. P. (1951) *Textbook of Psychiatry*. Trans. Brill, A. A. Dover Publications Inc., London.

Brend, W. A. (1938) *Traumatic Mental Disorders in Courts of Law*. William Heinemann, London.

111

Brill, N. Q. and Beebe, G. W. (1951) Follow-up study of psychoneuroses. *American Journal of Psychiatry* **108,** 417.

Brown, G. W. and Davidson, S. (1978) Social class, psychiatric disorder of mother and accidents to children. *Lancet* **i,** 378–381.

Dencker, S. J. (1958) A follow-up study of 128 closed head injuries in twins using co-twins as controls. *Acta Psychiatrica et Neurologica Scandinavica* **33,** Suppl. 123.

Dunbar, H. F. (1955) *Mind and Body.* Random House, New York.

Ferenczi, S. and Abraham, K. (1921) *Psychoanalysis and the War Neuroses.* G. E. Stehert and Co., New York.

Guttman, E. (1946) Late effects of closed head injuries: psychiatric observations. *Journal of Mental Science* **92,** 1.

Hillbom, E. (1960) After effects of brain injuries. *Acta Psychiatrica et Neurologica Scandinavica* **35,** Suppl. 142.

Hurst, A. F. (1916) *Medical Diseases of the War.* Edward Arnold, London.

Hurst, A. F. (1940) *Medical Diseases of War.* Edward Arnold, London.

Kardiner, A. and Spiegel, H. (1941) *War Stress and Neurotic Illness.* Paul B. Hoeber, London.

Keshavan, M. S., Channabasaranna, S. M., and Narayana Reddy, G. N. (1981) Post-traumatic psychiatric disturbances: patterns and predictors of outcome. *British Journal of Psychiatry* **138,** 157.

Klonoff, H. (1971) Head injuries in children—predisposing factors, accident conditions, accident proneness and sequelae. *American Journal of Public Health* **61,** 2405.

Kozol, H. L. (1945) Pre-traumatic personality and psychiatric sequelae of head injury. *Archives of Neurology and Psychiatry* **53,** 358.

Kral, V. A. (1951) Psychiatric observations under severe chronic stress. *American Journal of Psychiatry* **108,** 185.

Lewis, A. (1942) Discussion on differential diagnosis and treatment of post-concussional states. *Proceedings of the Royal Society of Medicine* **35,** 607.

Lewy, E. (1941) Compensation for war neurosis. *War Medicine* **1,** 887.

Lidvall, H. F., Linderoth, B. and Norlin, B. (1974) Causes of the post-concussional syndrome. *Acta Neurologica Scandinavica* **50,** Suppl. 56.

Lishman, W. A. (1978) *Organic Psychiatry.* Blackwells, London.

Merskey, H. and Trimble, M. R. (1979) Personality, sexual adjustment and brain lesions in patients with conversion symptoms. *American Journal of Psychiatry* **136,** 179.

Mitchell, S. W., Morehouse, C. R. and Keen, W. S. (1864) *Gunshot Wounds and other Injuries of Nerves.* Lippincott, Philadelphia.

Mott, F. W. (1919) *War Neuroses and Shell Shock.* Oxford Medical Publications, London.

Myers, C. S. (1940) *Shell-shock in France 1914–18.* Cambridge University Press, Cambridge.

Partington, M. W. (1960) The importance of accident proneness in the aetiology of head injuries in childhood. *Archives of Diseases in Childhood* **35,** 215.

112

Reusch, J. and Bowman, K. M. (1945) Prolonged post-traumatic syndromes following head injury. *American Journal of Psychiatry* **102**, 145.

Ross, T. A. (1941) *Lectures on War Neuroses*. Edward Arnold and Co., London.

Schmidt, C. W., Perlin, S., Townes, W., Fisher, R. S. and Shaffer, J. W. (1972) Characteristics of drivers involved in single car accidents. *Archives of General Psychiatry* **27**, 800.

Selzer, M. L., Rogers, J. E. and Kern, S. (1968) Fatal accidents: the role of psychopathology, social stress and acute disturbances. *American Journal of Psychiatry* **124**, 1028.

Shaw, L. and Sichel, H. S. (1971) *Accident Proneness. Research in the occurrence, causation and prevention of road accidents.* Pergamon, Oxford.

Sims, A. (1978) Hypotheses linking neuroses with premature mortality. *Psychological Medicine* **8**, 255.

Slater, E. (1943) The neurotic constitution. *Journal of Neurology and Psychiatry* **6**, 1.

Southward, E. E. (1919) *Shell Shock*. W. M. Leonard, Boston.

Symonds, C. P. (1937) Mental disorder following head injury. *Proceedings of the Royal Society of Medicine* **30**, 1081.

Symonds, C. P. (1943) The human response to flying stress. *British Medical Journal* **2**, 703.

Thomas, J. C. (1943) Neuroses in wartime. *Vancouver Medical Association* **19**, 136.

Thompson, G. N. (1965) Post-traumatic psychoneurosis—a statistical survey. *American Journal of Psychiatry* **121**, 1043.

Whitlock, F. A. (1971) *Death on the Road: a Study in Social Violence.* Tavistock Publications, London.

Whitlock, F. A., Stoll, J. R. and Rekhdahl, R. J. (1977) Crisis, life events and accidents. *Australian and New Zealand Journal of Psychiatry* **11**, 127.

CHAPTER 7

Variants and Nervous Shock

This book started with a discussion of railway spine and its relationship to the neuroses, and perhaps of necessity most of the studies referred to have been related to the field of head injuries and their consequences. However, a modern variant of the railway spine theme is seen in the condition referred to as the 'whiplash injury'. Although these injuries were actually first reported in pilots of catapult-assisted takeoff aircraft from aircraft carriers (a problem much diminished by supporting the pilot's head during takeoff), they came to prominence after World War II with the vast increase in motor traffic that occurred. Of all motor car accidents, 35% are the result of one vehicle driving into the back of another, with consequent unsupported sudden head movement of the person in the front car. The flexion is within physiological limits, but the extension is much greater than the normal range of approximately 45° and about one-fifth of passengers in rear-end collisions have significant injury as a result of this. Experimental studies, using brave volunteers, show that a force of 9 g at the neck can occur from a rear end impact of approximately 10 mph, and this is multiplied to 23 gs at the forehead. So-called acceleration injury of the head thus occurs without actual direct impact to the head. As after closed head injury, often following such an accident the patient presents with a variety of symptoms but on examination no neurological signs are to be detected. The symptoms are typical, and include headaches, dizziness, tinnitus, paraesthesiae, and pains in the neck and chest. Concussion is not usually reported, although some series suggest that up to 60% of patients have some evidence of concussion after such injury, with momentary loss of consciousness. The incidence of emotional disturbance in these patients is also high, up to 50% of patients developing an ensuing psychoneurotic illness (Gay and Abbot, 1953).

From the legal point of view certain things are clear. First, there is rarely a question of liability in these accidents, in that a driver who crashes into the back of another is inevitably at fault. In addition, many of the cases seem to involve the car in front being actually stationary, or travelling very slowly at the time of impact. In court, however, the same arguments that have been discussed before regarding the aetiology of post-traumatic neurosis are brought forward. The disagreement over the organic factors involved in producing the symptoms is of the same intensity, and the cry of malingering is often heard. However, in dealing with the problem of whiplash injuries there is also a dearth of studies on which to base opinions.

Gorman (1979) has pointed out that the hyperflexion which stretches the spinal cord can cause damage to a variety of structures including emerging spinal nerves. Since 10 % of normal people have a tight vertebral canal in the cervical region, the spinal cord is particularly at jeopardy from such injuries. In addition the vertebral artery can be markedly deformed by flexion, and the auditory and vestibular structures supplied by it may show objective signs of injury following whiplash, such as disturbance of tonic neck reflexes, nystagmus, and hearing loss at 4000 to 6000 Hz. In one reported autopsy, ligamentous and muscular tears were noted in the middle and lower cervical spine region.

Some follow-up studies of patients have been carried out. On the grounds that compensation itself may have been an important factor in producing symptoms, Gotten (1956) surveyed 100 patients following litigation settlement and reported that 88 were 'largely recovered'. He went on to comment:

'The fact that the symptoms did not adjust to treatment or that they at times would get worse, but improved after settlement of claims, cast doubt in our minds on the validity of the symptoms. . . .'

It is important to note, however, that in this series only 54 were free of troublesome symptoms, and 4 of 49 patients who received compensation and were satisfied with it, were still wearing a Thomas collar at follow-up.

Alternatively, McNab (1974) reported on a follow-up of 266 patients, two or more years following settlement. Of 145 that were examined, 121 continued to have symptoms, and he concluded that 'satisfactory conclusion of settlement or court action failed to relieve symptoms in 45 % of the group studied . . . the other published follow-ups show little variance in the type of end result'. The same author extended his observations in two directions. Clinically he was impressed by the fact that, in contrast to the above results, patients who face the back of the car at the time of the injury and experienced uncontrolled flexion of the neck had no ensuing pain, and that those involved in side collisions had a significantly smaller percentage of disabilities than those involved in collisions from the rear. In addition he used an experimental animal model of whiplash injuries to assess subsequent injury, and noted various muscular tears which were often associated with haematomas and haemorrhages, and disc injuries with tearing the anterior longitudinal ligament and separation of the disc from associated vertebra. He concluded:

'These experiments show that recognisable lesions can be produced. They show that the lesions can vary from being very minor injuries, such as a tear of the muscular fibres, to serious lesions, such as separation of the disc or damage to posterior joints.'

Toglia (1976) examined 309 patients with symptoms, especially dizziness following whiplash injuries. Using vestibular tests, including search for nystagmus with electronystagmography, he noted latent nystagmus in 29 % of patients, abnormal caloric tests in 57 % and rotatory test abnormalities in 51 %. He concluded that patients' subjective complaints were accompanied by detectable vestibular disturbance, even though more formal neurological examination may be normal.

Another mode of transport which has brought with it dangers and accidents, and thus similar sequelae, is the aeroplane. That flying itself could be stressful and provoke psychiatric symptoms has been recognized almost since the aeroplane was invented (Birley, 1920), and 'flying stress' became recognized as an entity related to the occupation. Symonds' (1943) investigation of psychiatric disorders in flying personnel has already been discussed. In that study he found that the incidence of neurosis was directly related to the amount of hazard encountered, being highest in night bombers and amongst rear gunners of heavy bombers. He supported the idea of a reciprocal relationship between stress and the predisposition to stress in the production of the final clinical symptoms and suggested that one of the most important elements in the stress which led to the neurosis was exposure to danger. This led to a state of fear which was persistent, and consequently led to the neurosis. He discussed the idea that fear could develop, and be persistent, after a danger had passed, and again some quantitative reciprocal relationship between stimulus and constitution existed. 'This tendency for fear to perseverate may be observed in many persons if the stimulus has been violent, but in relation to the stimuli of average intensity it is remarkable in certain individuals, suggesting an innate propensity to react in this manner.' He went on to give a case history which illustrated the point:

'Case 3 p-Oz, G.M., pilot aged 27, flying hours 240, operational hours on day bombers 100. This officer had since childhood been unduly sensitive to slights, easily depressed and lacking in confidence. His squadron suffered heavy casualties and eventually he was wounded in the leg on a sortie over the North Sea. He flew his damaged aircraft home but it blew up on landing. He won the George Medal for pulling his air-gunner out of the blazing wreckage. After two months in hospital he was physically fit to fly but was tense, anxious, depressed and self-reproachful. The illness here was clearly attributable to flying duties. Flying stress was rated as severe. Predisposition was moderate, non-flying stress nil.'

This case history demonstrates that people who survive a disaster, even when there is no head injury to themselves, are quite susceptible to the development of neurosis. This is similar to 'nervous shock' discussed by Page. Writing as he was about railway accidents, he could have been describing any of a number of accidents that occur to human beings in the course of their lives. He said:

'The suddenness of the accident, which comes without warning, or with a warning which only reveals the utter helplessness of the traveller, the loud noise, the hopeless confusion, the cries of those who are injured; these in themselves, and more especially if they occur at night or in the dark, are surely adequate to produce a profound impression on the nervous system.'

Although the concept of nervous shock may seem separate in some ways from that of the neurosis following actual physical injury, or head injury, the symptoms are often very similar, as may be the mechanism of their production, and legally it is an acceptable claim for damages, and has been upheld in court on many occasions. For example, in the case of Yates v. South Kirby Collieries (1910), a workman helped another who had been crushed beneath a fallen timber-prop, and the latter subsequently died. The man Yates developed symptoms, was unable to return to work and, was awarded compensation. Mr Justice Farewell said that: 'In my opinion nervous shock due to accident is as much personal injury due to accident as a broken leg.' Later in time, Lord Macmillan said in the case of *Hay* v. *Young* (1943):

'The crude view that the law should take cognizance only of physical injury resulting from actual impact has been discarded and it is now well-recognised that an action will lie for injury by shock sustained through the medium of the eye or the ear without direct contact. The distinction between the mental shock and bodily injury was never a scientific one. . . .'

Large sums of money have, in fact, been awarded for shock and subsequent neurosis, as in the case of *Hinz* v. *Berry* (1970), when a wife saw her husband being killed.

The legal consequences of 'nervous shock' are not only confined to compensation issues, as noted in a fascinating case study recently published by Parker (1980). He reported the case of Vince, one of monozygous twins born in Australia in 1933, and brought up in a strict fundamentalist Christian background. Both men went through uneventful schooling and married and prospered. However, Vince's life was dramatically changed by an accident when he was 42 years old, in which a truck that he was driving collided with a vehicle driven by a drunken man who failed to acknowledge a stop sign. The truck overturned and Vince and his two sons were trapped inside the cabin. Since petrol was flowing everywhere, he became anxious to the point of panic, fearing that they would all be burnt to death. In that accident his physical injuries were minimal, but following it he had to be admitted to a psychiatric unit for assessment and treatment. Then two years later he was involved in another accident in which his truck was speared by a long steel girder which fell from another vehicle travelling in front of him. Again, he did not sustain any significant physical injuries, but his anxiety symptoms returned with such severity that he was readmitted to the psychiatric hospital. Apparently everybody that knew him noted a dramatic change in his personality following the first accident, and in particular he was 'no longer the tolerant or forgiving Christian whom they knew, and little things would annoy him'. He became angry, irritable, and depressed, and noticeably more physically violent, particularly unusual since both twins had always held strong views about expressing anger and would even get somebody else to kill an animal for them if it was necessary. In 1978, three years after his first accident and while still receiving psychiatric treatment, he murdered his wife by strangling her and his daughter by stabbing her with a bread-knife, following which he tried unsuccessfully to kill himself. Of great importance in this case history is his identical twin brother who was also available for examination. Intellectual and personality differences were noted between the two twins on assessment after the accidents in contrast to their very similar prior development. When the background details of the two brothers were examined carefully, Parker felt it was 'reasonable to conclude that Vince would today be the same well-controlled personality as his co-twin Ernest, but for the two life-threatening accidents'. In this case his neurosis developed without evidence of brain damage or trauma and without any compensation, since this was never considered in either accident.

The phenomenon of nervous shock is observed frequently in those who are involved in, and survive, major disasters. Such events, of course, have been known to affect mankind since the beginnings of recorded history and, presumably, existed prior to that. Their effects on the mental state of people involved, however, have only in recent times been studied systematically. An example of the way a disaster is experienced is William James's (1911) own account of an earthquake:

'First I personified the earthquake as a permanent individual entity. It came, moreover, directly to *me*. It stole in behind my back, and once inside the room, had me all to itself, and could manifest itself convincingly. Animus and intent were never more present in any human action, nor did any human activity ever more definitely point back to a living agent as its source and origin. All whom I consulted on the point agreed as to this feature in their experience; "it expressed intention", "it was vicious", "it was bent on destruction", "it wanted to show its power", or what-not . . . the perception of it as a living agent was irresistible. It had an overpowering dramatic convincingness.'

Among the studies of actual disaster victims the results collected by Leopold and Dillon (1963) are significant for the theme of this book. They studied the survivors of an accident in which a gasoline tanker called Mission San Francisco collided with the Elna 11—a freighter, in the Delaware River. The collision produced a series of explosions in which the captain of the Mission, all three deck officers, five crewmen, and the pilot were killed. The engineers and crew at the stern of the boat, however, survived but were 'tossed about and shaken'. Of the 45 men on board the boat, 35 lived as did all 23 of the Elna crew. The authors examined 36 of the total survivors and followed 25 of them for $3\frac{1}{2}$ to 4 years. The majority were veterans of long service at sea: 26 had served more than 11 years, and conditions of danger and threat were not unknown to them. Only 9 had a previous psychiatric history. Little physical injury was apparent immediately after the disaster, but psychological complaints were reported by 26 patients, especially nervousness, tension, and anxiety. Less frequent complaints were of restlessness, depression, and preoccupation with the details of the accident. A small number of patients were quite devastated by their experience, and four were admitted to hospital for psychiatric treatment. However, the later follow-up of these patients revealed further psychopathology. The authors reported:

'The interim medical histories in themselves attested to the extent the emotional suffering these men had endured. At least 26 received psychiatric intervention and 12 were hospitalised. The somatic involvements reported in 1960/61, more numerous than those for 1957, were largely musculoskeletal, the majority involving the muscles of the back and the neck. Although considerable muscle spasm was found, the presence of neurological or bony disease could not be confirmed.'

In addition, over half the patients examined at follow-up complained of continuous and sometimes disabling headaches. Although two-thirds of the men went back to work in three months, only 12 of the sample were actually able to return to sea with regular employment, the rest working at a level below their previous experience. Four never returned to sea at any time, and 12 returned for only a short period. The authors went on to develop a 'regressive score', which was essentially a numerical score of the change in psychological status between their examinations, which they then correlated with clinical factors. The highest incidence of regression was found in a group of 12 men who returned to sea but were forced to leave their job after return, or who returned but were unable to work adequately.

These findings are significant for understanding the problem of post-traumatic neurosis. Thus, unlike many of the other studies of disasters, which tend to look at catastrophes which occur in settled communities, the authors of this study took what might be termed 'disaster in the microcosm'. The elements of litigation were diminished, in that the seamen would have gained compensation quite easily since they only had to show that injury was suffered during service, and not because of it, in order to obtain recompense. In addition, the majority of these men had apparently relatively stable premorbid personalities. The authors concluded:

'Neither the intellectual awareness of the potential dangers they faced, particularly in terms of explosions, nor emotional attachment to the sea, was sufficient to be of value to these men when catastrophe overtook them. One must wonder what prevented prior knowledge from being of protective value. It appears that repeated performance of a dangerous occupation dulls the capacity for anticipation, fearful or otherwise of disaster. . . . When injury does occur the victim is unprepared to cope with the resultant alterations of self.'

They felt that the nature of an accident, especially its suddenness, was more significant in determining the outcome from the psychological point of view than was the premorbid personality. Litigation and compensation issues were not considered important in their study since many of those who abandoned the sea obtained alternative less remunerative and less prestigious occupations, but to most of them the sea represented a way of life as well as means of earning a living. The authors commented:

'Yet without the prime factor of monetary gain these exhibited psychological damage patterns comparable to those so often described as litigation anxiety, compensation neurosis, and in other pejorative terms.'

The psychological sequelae of disasters have recently been reviewed by Kinston and Rosser (1974). Of the impact of the disaster itself they say: 'The myth of personal invulnerability, so powerful in the threat phase, suffers a sudden reversal . . . the individual is actually encountering death.' They pointed out the dearth of studies dealing with the long-term consequences of stress, but particularly pinpointed those which showed that there is a much higher mortality and morbidity rate in post-war years for prisoners of war than in, for example, combat veterans. In addition, there is a higher incidence of sequelae in people who were interned in Japanese camps as opposed to European camps. The so-called 'concentration camp syndrome' is now recognized (Eitinger, 1961). One group called it 'repatriation neurosis' (Helweg-Larsen et al. 1952) and reported 75% of ex-prisoners they investigated to have neurotic symptoms, especially restlessness, fatigue, irritability, and vegetative nervous symptoms. Eitinger's study of 100 patients who had been imprisoned included 93 who 'could be called fairly even, harmonious and well-balanced personalities, without any special inter-personal contact difficulties or neurotic traits'. His main findings were nervousness, irritability, restlessness, memory deficits, dysphoria, and emotional instability, impairment of sleep, anxiety, and headaches—which affected over 50% of the sample. It is relevant to note that in Eitinger's series, positive neurological findings occurred in 88 cases. In that the camp experience often involved severe weight loss, encephalitis, typhus, and head injuries, he said:

'Our figures appear then to confirm the assumption that organic brain changes produced by the various traumatic situations reported . . . form the basis of the concentration camp syndrome. . . . On the whole, it is only the intensity, both in quality and quantity, of the concentration camp stress which seems to be decisive for the severity of both the concentration camp syndrome and the organic brain syndrome.'

They thus implicated organic changes of a mechanical and perhaps toxic nature in the aetiology of the neurosis.

Kinston and Rosser in their review article stated that the syndrome 'closely resembles post-traumatic neurosis'. Similar results have been found by others (Strøm, 1968), although the relationship between the organic brain changes and the affective disorders is not always reported so clearly. While the extent of the organic damage seems related to physical trauma, especially head trauma, in other studies the affective changes better correlated with the amount of anxiety suffered. More recently, Klonoff et al. (1976) have assessed the problem with a follow-up study 30 years after imprisonment. They compared a high stress group (Japanese internees), with a low stress group (European internees). This study reported neuropsychological impairment in 35.5% of the former and 19.0% of the latter, and psychiatric illness in 51.5% of the former and 28.6% of the latter. The low-stress subjects who had been interned for more than two years, showed a significantly greater neuropsychological impairment in most cases than those low-stress subjects who had been interned for less than two years. Fifty-one per cent of the high-stress group and 11.9% of the low-stress group had physical/neurological impairments. Their suggestion was that stress had long-term effects dependent on the nature and duration of the stress conditions, and that there occurred important neuro-psychological and neurological sequelae.

Minski (1978) made a similar distinction between Far East prisoners of war and ex-German prisoners of war in relation to the consequent psychiatric disability. He suggested that in the former group the outstanding feature was extreme tension, as if they were living on the edge of a precipice, with associated irritability and aggression. Only a minority of his own series had constitutional factors to predispose to neurosis, although most were conscientious and obsessional. The prisoners were kept by the Japanese under constant threat of death, although their own attitude to death became detached, and remained so after release. Their nervous symptoms began to trouble them many years after the end of the war, although it was clear that they underwent personality changes on account of their experiences, from which they never recovered.

The similarity of the medical sequelae of survival of disaster to post-traumatic neurosis commented on by Kinston and Rosser has also been noted in reports from the aftermath of the Aberfan disaster, the Bristol floods, and, more recently, the Buffalo Creek disaster.

The Aberfan disaster occurred in 1966. A high tip situated above the mining community of Aberfan collapsed and engulfed the town, resulting in the deaths of 116 children and 28 adults. Following this accident, direction from all over the world was focused on the small town, and this publicity itself brought further problems to the affected victims, likened perhaps to the attention received by the victim of an industrial accident. One observer commented:

'The news media gave intensive coverage to all that was going on and hardened attitudes or opinions, that might ordinarily have been fleeting, into something more permanent . . . many people in Aberfan became very hostile to the press. . . . It soon became apparent that those involved had a need to express aggression against some official body or group, such as the Coal Board, local authority, the government etc.' (Lacey, 1972)

A high incidence of neurosis was reported following the disaster and, in particular, the children were markedly affected. The latter is an important observation in terms of compensation issues, since it might be expected that children would have been unaware of such issues, and even if they were aware of them, were less likely to have understood them.

Bennet (1970) described the effects on the health of the local community of the Bristol floods in July 1968. Five inches of rain fell in 12 hours, and 3000 houses, shops, and other properties were damaged by the flood. The water in many cases reached the ceilings of the ground-floor rooms, and, after it subsided, left everything it had touched covered by a fine layer of stinking mud. Bennet compared the incidence of medical attendances in patients affected by the floods with a control group and found that the former were increased such that more of the flooded group went several times to their GPs and hospital in the 12 months after the event compared with the year before the floods. This was more pronounced in those who had experienced deeper flooding. The mortality in the experimental group rose 50% in the subsequent year, and among the flooded men 33% reported new 'physical' symptoms, and among the women 18% new psychiatric pathology. Such rises were much greater than in controls. Bennet compared these results to other work which has shown a rise in surgery attendance, morbidity, and mortality following bereavement.

The community at Buffalo Creek, West Virginia, was studied perhaps more intensely than the survivors from Bristol and Aberfan. In Buffalo Creek in 1972 a slag dam gave way and unleashed a deluge of water and mud on Buffalo Creek Valley, killing 125 people and leaving a further 4000 homeless. Some 654 survivors subsequently began legal action against the company that owned the dam (Titchener and Kapp, 1976). 'A traumatic neurotic syndrome was diagnosed in more than 80% of the survivor-plaintiffs. . . .' Of the 224 children survivor-plaintiffs most were found to be significantly emotionally impaired (Newman, 1976). The medico-legal aspects of the Buffalo Creek disaster have been recorded and were revealing. The outcome was of settlement for $13.5 million dollars, $6 million of which was for psychological damages (Titchener and Kapp, 1976). The coal company apparently employed an independent psychiatrist, who was a physician with a primary interest in neurosurgery. He, along with a psychologist in training, examined the cases, and reached the decision that the survivors had only transient situational disturbances which would abate soon after the disaster. However, when he re-examined them eighteen months later and found they still had the same psychological disturbances, he was led to presume that these people were suffering primarily from pre-existing illnesses (Stern, 1976). The plaintiff's physicians indicated that the psychiatric damage was solely caused by the disaster. They went further and insisted that even people not present at the disaster, but merely residents who suffered loss and subsequent psychiatric sequelae should be compensated. The courts agreed with this and individually each survivor received between $7000 and $10,000 after legal fees were deducted.

Observations on survivors of disasters have now been recorded on a number of different occasions after, for example, shipwreck

(Henderson and Bostock, 1977) and hijacking (*Time*, 1977). The clinical presentation of the victims is remarkably similar, and recognition of the ensuing neurotic illness is well recorded. Some governments now acknowledge that the psychological sequelae are profound, and centres are sometimes established to deal with victims immediately following the event, in an attempt to prevent the later complications. Several authors suggest that if early psychiatric intervention had been available for the prisoners of war, the sequelae would have been prevented (e.g. Minski, 1978), although the evidence for this is not well documented. Psychotherapy, individual or group, psychoanalysis, and abreaction have all had their advocates, especially aimed at the relief of guilt, tension, and grief. The American psychiatrists in particular have had considerable experience in this field, as a consequence of both the Korean and Vietnam wars. Baker (1975) noted the principles applied in treatment to be 'those of proximity, immediacy, and expectancy'. The model was that of crisis intervention, with adequate sedation, and recognition that fatigue and fear were prominent requiring 'rest, sleep, food and respite from stress'. Recently Stöfsel (1980) has reported the results of intervention and aftercare following the hijacking of a train in the north of Holland by South Moluccans. Ninety-six passengers were taken, although 42 were soon released. Forty-nine were freed after three weeks by the army in an attack which killed two of the passengers and six of the Moluccans. The survivors were given the earliest opportunity to talk about their emotional experiences, and their fears about after effects. Short-term problems were mainly tension, insomnia, fear, and phobias which were seen in most of those followed. Long-term effects appearing after four weeks occurred in two-ihirds, and included irritability, fear, phobias, vague physical complaints, insomnia, and feelings of insecurity. In 85 % these feelings were new experiences, and only 15 % had noted the same symptoms prior to the hijack. Active intervention by the research team seemed to be of value to the victims and 'the negative after effects were more serious when the event was eliminated from consciousness during the first weeks after release, or conversely, when the victim had been too intensely preoccupied with it.' They recommended the setting up of special centres which victims of violent acts could contact for information and professional help, and the training of specialized personnel to deal with such problems.

'Nervous shock' then, is a widely reported disorder, recognized by the courts, with symptoms indistinguishable from post-traumatic neurosis. The premorbid personality may play a role in its production, but it seems, from the evidence presented, related more to the disaster or event itself, rather than the personality involved. As Kinston and Rosser (1974) have put it:

'Following the Black Death there was an age marked by misery, depression, anxiety and a general sense of impending doom. The plague was a chronic frightening threat about which nothing could be done. However, today we both expect and demand survival; society admits the narcissistic entitlement, the right to survive.'

Reported law cases

Hay v. Young (1943) A.C. 9Z
Hinz v. Berry (1970) Z Q.B. 40
Yates v. South Kirby Collieries (1910) 2 K.B. 538.

References

Baker, S. L. (1975) Military psychiatry. In *Comprehensive Textbook of Psychiatry*, Vol. 2. Ed. Freedman, A. M., Kaplan, H. I. and Sadock, B. J. Williams and Wilkins, Baltimore.

Bennet, G. (1970) Bristol floods in 1968. *British Medical Journal* **3**, 454.

Birley, J. (1920) Principles of medical science as applied to military aviation. *Lancet* **i**, 1147, 1205, 1251.

Eitinger, L. (1961) Pathology of the concentration camp syndrome. *Archives of General Psychiatry* **5**, 371.

Gay, J. R. and Abbott, K. H. (1953) Common whiplash injuries of the neck. *Journal of the American Medical Association* **152**, 1698.

Gorman, W. F. (1979) Whiplash: fictive or factual. *Bulletin of the American Academy of Psychiatry and the Law* **7**, 245–248.

Gotten, N. (1956) Survey of one hundred cases of whiplash injury after settlement of litigation. *Journal of the American Medical Association* **162**, 865.

Helweg-Larsen, P., Hoffmeyer, H., Kieler, J., Thaysen, E. H., Thaysen, J. H., Thygesen, P. and Wulff, M. H. (1952) Famine disease in German concentration camps, complications and sequels with special reference to tuberculosis, mental disorders and social consequences. *Acta Medica Scandinavica* **144**, Suppl. 274, 3.

Henderson, S. and Bostock, T. (1977) Coping behaviour after shipwreck. *British Journal of Psychiatry* **131**, 15.

Hoffmeyer, H., Kieler, J., Thaysen, J. H., Thygesen, P. and Wulff, M. H. (1952) Famine disease in German concentration camps. *Acta Psychiatrica Scandinavica* Suppl. 83.

126

James, W. (1911) On some mental effects of the earthquake. In *Memories and Studies*. Longmans Green, New York.

Kinston, W. and Rosser, R. (1974) Disaster: effects on mental and physical state. *Journal of Psychosomatic Research* **18**, 437.

Klonoff, H., McDougall, G., Kramer, P. and Horgan, J. (1976) The neuropsychological, psychiatric and physical effects of prolonged and severe stress: 30 years after. *Journal of Nervous and Mental Disease* **163**, 246.

Lacey, G. N. (1972) Observations on Aberfan. *Journal of Psychosomatic Research* **16**, 257.

Leopold, R. L. and Dillon, H. (1963) Psychoanatomy of a disaster. *American Journal of Psychiatry* **119**, 913.

McNab, I. (1974) The whiplash syndrome. *Clinical Neurosurgery* **20**, 232

Minski, L. (1978) Far East prisoners of war. *Bethlem and Maudsley Gazette*, Winter Edition.

Newman, C. J. (1976) Children of disaster. Clinical observations at Buffalo Creek. *American Journal of Psychiatry* **133**, 306.

Parker, N. (1980) Personality change following accidents. The report of a double murder. *British Journal of Psychiatry* **137**, 401.

Stern, G. M. (1976) From chaos to responsibility. *American Journal of Psychiatry* **133**, 301.

Stöfsel, W. (1980) Psychological sequelae in hostages and the aftercare. *Danish Medical Bulletin* **27**, 239.

Strøm, A. (1968) Quoted in Lancet Leader 'Late effects of torture'. *Lancet* **ii**, 721.

Symonds, C. P. (1943) The human response to flying stress. *British Medical Journal* **2**, 703.

Time (1977) After the rescue: hijack therapy. 20th June 1977.

Titchener, J. L. and Kapp, F. T. (1976) Family and character change at Buffalo Creek. *American Journal of Psychiatry* **133**, 295.

Toglia, J. U. (1976) Acute flexion–extension injury of the neck. *Neurology* **26**, 808.

CHAPTER 8

Some Medico-legal Aspects

It is not the intention of this chapter to give advice about etiquette in court or even information about procedure. Much of this can be found in Brend's book (Brend, 1938). It is intended, however, to discuss some of the differences that arise between one medical opinion and another and the reasons for the discrepancy and, in addition, to highlight some of the difficulties the legal mind has when it comes across the medical mind.

Anyone in medical practice may be asked to provide an assessment of post-traumatic symptoms in a patient, and some, especially at neurological hospitals, are called on frequently. The bulk of the practice comes from sequelae of car accidents and injury at work. Anyone injured is entitled under the law to take action against another where negligence can be established. With regard to industrial injury, the law has expanded considerably over the years in this country and many others on account of the various Workmen's Compensation Acts, the first of which in England was in 1897.

Prior to this there was little an injured workman could do in order to seek redress from an employer. There were well-known defences which were open to the employers' representatives, which often led to the defeat of any litigation. Particularly important in this respect was the fact that if a workman was injured as a result of his own negligence, he was deemed responsible for the accident. The successive Acts removed the association of fault and liability, and made it necessary only that the workman prove that he suffered an injury in the course of his employment and, of course, there came with this the statutory obligation of the employer to pay any compensation that was awarded. The workman's own negligence also became disregarded, and in the event of serious disablement or death, not even obvious misconduct or abrogation of the rules could be used as a defence.

While earlier acts excluded domestic and menial servants from the definition of workman, the 1925 Act was almost universal in application, referring to any person working under apprenticeship or contract with an employer.

It was clear that much was wrong with the original Acts and they underwent some twenty or more amendments in the first 50 years after they were enacted. As a commentator said:

'One reflects with wonder at the consternation of the legislators circa 1897 could they but have had a peep through half a century of the laws they were formulating . . . either (they) had been unduly optimistic and badly informed or they had failed to attach significant importance to the psychological and other effects of the passing of such legislation' (Slater, 1946).

Thus what happened was demonstrated amongst others by Collie in his book on malingering, and his figures have already been quoted. These essentially showed the increase in non-fatal industrial accidents which ensued in the years following legislation. Although a Home Office report in 1912 suggested that the increase was probably related to the fact that, as the Act became better known, more workmen stayed away for injury which could previously have meant their struggling on at work, Collie himself suggested that it was the compensation that was responsible. The illogicality of the Act was pointed out by him thus:

'It is hardly to be expected of human nature that a man whose injury incapacitates him for 12 days, thereby entitling him to five days' compensation, will return to work on the 13th day, when, by postponing his return for two days, he will become entitled to 14 days' pay.'

A similar point was made by others with regard to war neuroses. Lewy (1941) felt that the neuroses were maintained by the compensation, in that the latter became part of secondary gain. He said the state thus 'makes itself guilty of tempting the neurotic person to become chronically ill, for the rent is, so to speak, a reward for chronic invalidism and a temptation which only a few people would be able to resist'. Kalinowsky (1950) reported that an expert testimony in Germany in 1926 led to a High Court decision to the effect that 'when a disability is caused by the patient's idea of being sick, or by more or less conscious wishes, the preceding traumatic experience is not the essential cause of his disability, even if the traumatic experience elicited the idea of being sick or raised the hope of financial compensation'. He reported that this decision led to a decrease in the numbers of post-traumatic nervous disorders in Germany, a decrease which continued through World War II.

One solution to the problems raised by compensation acts then would be to deny any compensation for post-traumatic neurosis at all and such action has been suggested both for war and for peace-time post-traumatic illness. This, however, would be humanely impossible, and unacceptable to institutions such as trade union organizations. Another solution would be to modify the way compensation is paid. Thus, Lewy suggested that a lump sum rather than weekly or monthly payments should be adopted. While the former is the usual case with war neurosis, it was not always adopted with compensation claims related to civilian injuries. Thus the 1906 and 1925 Acts recommended weekly payments in compensation, although there were provisions originally in the Acts for the employer to apply for a lump sum settlement after six months. The idea, presumably, was that the lump sum could then be invested and converted into a life annuity.

The Acts never clearly held to their original intentions, and became, as all legislation seems inevitably to do, more complex with technical loopholes that invalidated some of their purpose. Thus, even if an injured workman managed to find his way successfully to court, and survived the ordeal of trial with all that it involved, there was no guarantee that the awarded compensation would, in fact, be paid. The firm involved may have gone bankrupt, and in any case even before all this, many employees actually bargained away their legal rights for a lump sum payment, which was then presumably spent unwisely. The Acts actually spread much ill feeling and distrust between workers and employers, and were thought to be harmful to industrial relations.

The Beveridge Committee was set up during World War II specifically to look into a wide range of social security benefits, which included Workmen's Compensation. As a result of that committee's report, the Industrial Injuries Fund was set up. This fund, run by a state department, was supported by small contributions from both the employed and the employers, and was fundamentally a compulsory insurance scheme against industrial accidents. Claims were, and still are, made to this fund, and not to an individual employer, thus removing the main disadvantage of the old system. Under this new scheme, liability was not particularly at issue, and the main point was whether or not personal injury by accident arose 'out of and in the course of employment'. Even then, injury due to 'serious or wilful misconduct' of workmen, which had previously, except in very severe cases, been a case for disallowing compensation, became irrelevant. In addition to this, the Beveridge Report also led to the abolition of the system of lump sum payments, and in contradiction to some opinions expressed above, suggested that such payments 'led a man to prolong an incapacity and disturb his social life'.

The position at the present time is that claims for industrial accidents are assessed initially by a civil servant, who allows or disallows the claim. Settlements are referred to as injury benefit and consist of weekly payments on an all or nothing basis for 26 weeks. Appeal to a local tribunal, presided over by a barrister or solicitor, is permitted. If the period of disability is likely to be longer than 26 weeks then disablement benefit can be allowed. This is assessed either after receiving the short-term benefit or without it, and is awarded as a percentage disability, dependent on the amount of disablement suffered. This is usually assessed by a Medical Board, and is made for a fixed period, which may be life. Unless the sums are very small, weekly payments are made.

An important principle introduced into the 1906 Act was that any right to compensation was made independent of any claim to recover either at Common Law, or under the Employers' Liability Act. Thus, anyone has the right under Common Law to claim damages against a person whose negligence has caused injury which leads, in many cases, to parallel claims operating. In contrast to the state system, the Common Law awards lump sum payments for damages.

Several persistent problems arise during the medico-legal assessment of compensation issues—for example, interpreting the actual relationship of the accident to the symptoms with which the claimant presents. In addition, there is the problem of assessing damages when there is some pre-existing injury or 'vulnerability'. On the first point the law is fairly clear. Generally it adopts what has been called the 'but for' test

'If the damage would not have happened but for a particular fault, then that fault is the cause of the damage; if it would have happened just the same, fault or no fault, the fault is not the cause of the damage.' (Jolowicz et al., 1971)

Now this is very pragmatic and has a certain amount of logic to it; however, it often is at odds with medical thinking where causality is rarely thought to be determined by a single event and is usually seen as multifactorial. This point is one which frequently leads to much confusion and conflicting evidence, and differences between doctors and lawyers. The law seems to be assessing the straw that breaks the camel's back, and in many cases different doctors can be brought forward to implicate different straws. Two often-quoted examples of the 'but for' principle are as follows. In the case of *Cutler* v. *Vauxhall Motors Limited* (1971), the plaintiff grazed his right ankle in an accident but subsequently developed, at the site of the graze, a varicose ulcer. Of couse, varicosities had been present prior to the injury, but the injury actually resulted in the development of the ulcer. Thus, there followed an operation and a request for compensation for loss of earnings and pain associated with the operation. The trial judge, and the Court of Appeal, disallowed this on account of the fact that the varicosity *per se* was unconnected with the accident. Here, the 'but for' test indicated that the varicosities would have worsened anyway, and would have therefore needed operation at some time. One judge, however, at the appeal, dissented on the grounds that what was essentially a probability had been converted into a certainty, a view some may have sympathy with. However, the appeal was clearly disallowed on the 'but for' principle.

In the case of *Baker* v. *Willoughby* (1970), the plaintiff had suffered a leg injury and was forced to take up a new job. In the new job he was the victim of an armed robbery and suffered further injury to his already injured leg, and finally the leg had to be amputated. The 'but for' test here would suggest that liability of the defendant who caused the first injury was limited to the loss suffered before the second injury, which was the decision of the Court of Appeal. This is diagrammatically represented in Figure 8.1. The original accident occurred at x, and the plaintiff's assets are represented by the unbroken line. His losses are thus a, until the second accident at y, when n represents his actual position after the second injury, and m the expected position if he had only one injury. Thus $a + b$ are the losses he would have sustained following only one injury. However, the argument then is over who should be liable for b, the perpetrator of the first or second injury (Ogus, 1973). Lord Pearson, in the House of Lords, observed that the Court of Appeal argument led to manifest injustice, especially since it was not possible to sue the robbers. Accordingly the defendant was liable for the full extent of the injury (a and b), without reduction or limitation on account of the subsequent injury.

There is often great difficulty in reality in demonstrating a cause and effect relationship between accident and injury symptoms, and usually all that can be shown is some statistical relationship of increased probability between two factors, certain proof being unattainable. Since

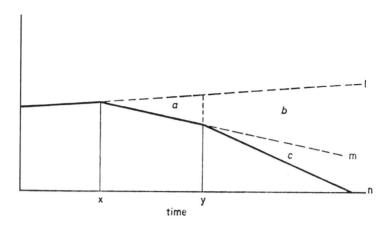

Figure 8.1 Causation and remoteness (from Ogus, 1973)

the medical consequences of injury require full knowledge of the aetiology and pathogenesis of subsequent medical disorders for full understanding of this relationship, and because there is little definitive knowledge of the origins of neurosis, it is not surprising that proof of the relationship between trauma and consequent neurosis is often a matter of vigorous argument. The fact that causality in law has a different emphasis from scientific causality leads to the illogical position that although cause–effect relationships are theoretically universal, juridical causation differs from one country to the next, implying that causality is relative to the country in which a person lives and not related to natural phenomena.

In determining whether or not a particular symptom is caused by a particular event, attention is always paid to the temporal factor. For this the law uses what is termed the 'foreseeability test' and 'the doctrine of remoteness'. Foreseeability, namely the loss such that a reasonable man could foresee resulting from an event, has been used in the courts to determine the existence of liability, rather than the quantum of compensation, thus delimiting the kind of harm for which damages are recoverable, rather than the extent of that harm. The 'doctrine of remoteness' is an attempt to distinguish events associated with, and events unassociated with, an accident. The criteria for this test is whether the consequences are or are not too remote from an initial cause to be considered. Bacon's maxim is often quoted: 'In jure non remota causa sed proxima spectatus.' However, this is not very scientific, and is essentially meaningless since, for example, the concept that tidal motion is related to the movement of the moon would be considered inappropriate by it, as indeed the idea was when Kepler originally put it forward. As Jolowicz *et al.* (1971) state:

'To a certain point the common law does touch on metaphysics. But no test of remoteness of causation put forward by Anglo-American courts would satisfy any metaphysician. On the other hand no test suggested by metaphysicians would be of any practical use to lawyers.'

As another legal commentator has it:

'Causation is to be understood as the man in the street and not as either the scientist or the metaphysician would understand it.'

'The trial of an action for damage is not a scientific inquest into a mixed sequence of phenomena, or an historical investigation of the chapter of events . . . it is a practical enquiry.' (Jolowicz *et al.*, 1971):

This again highlights the main differences between medical and legal thinking. Thus, doctors generally try to think scientifically and, as has just been noted, the rules of science are not the rules of courtroom. It seems unwise to bring in what the man in the street thinks, because very often the man in the street is incorrect, linking in a causal way things which scientifically have been shown to be non-causal. Perhaps nowhere is this more common than when linking accidents to subsequent medical symptoms. The presentation to doctors with cancer of the breast or multiple sclerosis within a few weeks of some minor injury is very common, and the two are often causally linked in the patient's mind. However, to date, from the scientific point of view, causality in problems such as these has never been determined. As Kräupl Taylor (1979) has recently summed it up:

'In modern theories, the principles of causality are no longer linked to deterministic postulates of inexorable bonds between cause and effect, but to postulates of energy transmissions and transformations.'

From the point of view of clinical psychiatry, logical relations are usually only those of 'weak implication', and at the philosophical level the proposition that all events have causes is neither provable nor refutable (Bebbington, 1980).

The difficulty is that the law is not interested in science, but in precedents. Lawyers, in their arguments, tend to employ deductive logic, whereas doctors use inductive methods, referring from the particular to the general. The law, in taking as its starting-point tradition and precedent is, of course, in direct opposition to the scientific mode of thinking, since both are highly anti-scientific. This must be one factor that has led the law to be particularly slow in adopting new ideas and understanding in the light of advancing scientific knowledge, seen most clearly in the field of psychiatric illness. However, lawyers are not alone in failing to alter their ideas, and many doctors also do not use available knowledge in an attempt to understand psychiatric disability, which in a trial relating to post-traumatic neurosis is a further source of conflict and misunderstanding.

Another difficulty between doctors and lawyers arises from ideological differences on the issue of freedom and will. Many doctors, especially since the more widespread understanding and acceptance of psychological influences that control behaviour and motivation, see the concept of free will only as relative to an individual's environmental and biological circumstances. For the lawyer it is assumed a person is free to act in one way or another, irrespective of the circumstances in which he finds himself. While, of course, the law is prepared to recognize insanity, the concept of sanity is based on intellect and comprehension, which is thought somehow to become altered in madness. This concept, of mind equating to reason, ignores much of modern psychology and psychiatry, and leads to conflicts between physicians and lawyers, the latter still struggling with an out-of-date framework in which to fit their ideas. Cartesian dualism, the concept that mind and body exist as two separate entities, with different frames of reference, pervades such discussions leading to problems of understanding. The two conflicting trends of explanation for post-traumatic neurosis outlined in this book, namely psychological or organic, reflect such dualism. Cicero's suggestion that the law should ask not *si insanus sed si furiosus est* indicates that these problems are by no means new. As Ellard (1970) has pointed out: 'It may be more profitable to consider what a symptom means than to try to determine how aware its owner is of his own mental processes.'

In the application of the legal principles outlined above, other problems also arise. It could be argued, for example, that the subsequent psychological state of the patient following an accident was an independent event, as happened in the German High Court. The appropriate legal maxim here is the *novus actus interveniens*. Thus, a pathological state of mind arises because, for example, the injured person broods on the accident, and the patient makes himself ill. In the case of *Pearson* v. *Pimms & Sons Ltd* a girl lost the end of her little finger and half of the ring finger of the right hand. After a period of time her employers applied to stop compensation payments and she was considered fit for work. The judge agreed, as it was not a sufficient answer for her to say she felt nervous at working the same machine again, and medical evidence indicated she was fit for work except with regard to her fear. The judge asserted that she might always be shy of the machine, and was she then to go on receiving compensation forever?

Likewise an employer is not liable to pay compensation to an employee simply because the latter thinks he is ill. However, this leads often to contradictory opinions, with considerable verbal confusion. For example, in one cited case, a man received injury, did not work and applied for compensation due to nervousness. The judge said:

'This is a typical neurasthenic case from the legal point of view. If the law be that the average reasonable man is allowed to stay away from work on account of nervousness, this case will be upset, and this very person, who fancies himself unable to work, will continue to draw a pension from the rest of the community, who will have to pay. I do not think this is the meaning of the Workman's Compensation Act.'

In another, where the problem was similar, we learn the judge stated of a plaintiff (Collie, 1933):

'It was important to remember that no-one says that is a malingerer. . . . The loss of will-power is just as much the result of the accident as any objective symptoms would be. . . . He is not a malingerer, but an honest man suffering from loss of will-power, due to the accident. . . .'

A further complication is that it is possible to suggest, as some authors already quoted have done, that post-traumatic neurosis can be distinguished from compensation neurosis, on the grounds that the latter are always associated with compensation. The compensation itself thus becomes a *novus actus interveniens*, and in a circular way, will invalidate the whole of the claim. While this position is rarely adopted, it is clear that, logically, it should be taken into account.

Pre-existing vulnerability is another factor which is often not considered in law, but which doctors are nearly always very much aware of. Thus, it is well known that it is not permissible to plead mitigation from damages if a person with an abnormally thin skull or unusually brittle bones has an injury from accident which is far greater than would be expected. It is an adage that the railway company must take passengers as they find them, complete with their disabilities and idiosyncrasies, and so too must any employer. While this may seem unfair to defendants, it is the method adopted by the courts, and it has led to the search for techniques to screen out those people who are liable to develop a neurosis at times of stress. While such methods do not have wide application in the industrial field to date, they may do in the future, particularly if the costs of compensation escalate. A practice of screening individuals for physical deficits which might later on become a source of a compensation claim already occurs. Some industries, where for example claims are made for deafness resulting from industrial noise, medically examine potential employees, and will not take on people with hearing deficits. Although this may seem hard on those with a degree of deafness, it makes for good economic sense from the industry's point of view.

The law, in spite of its shortcomings over understanding modern concepts of psychiatric illness, does however clearly recognize neurotic disorder and, in particular, the concept of the post-traumatic neuroses, and it is fair to say that neurosis is accepted as a recognized mental illness with its own characteristics and symptoms. Thus one well-known legal textbook gives a description which shows far greater understanding than many contemporary medical texts. Munkman (1980) states:

'The network of nerves throughout the body—partly bringing in various sensations, partly "motor" nerves controlling movement—is a physical system running through the spinal cord back to the brain, the central nervous system. Any physical injury to any part of this system, especially any brain injury, is a matter for the neurologist. Neurotic illnesses do also affect the central nervous system because the emotions, fear, anxiety etc. are brain functions. Also they may spread out to the external nervous system, producing, for example, hysterical paralysis. What we encounter here is wear and tear from the inside of the system, producing disordered working, hence neurosis is often described as "functional" rather than organic. But no doubt long-term malfunctioning also produces physical changes in parts of the brain or its chemistry . . .'.

However, the possibility that neurosis can be evoked by injury is obviously often not recognized and, as pointed out, patients so afflicted are often termed malingerers. The term 'post-traumatic neurosis' begs the question. Mr Justice Winn, in the trial of *James* v. *Woodall Duckham Construction* (1969) said:

'I would have ventured to think that no neurosis can properly be called a "traumatic" neurosis unless there is a continuous chain of causation between the trauma and the neurosis. The fact that a neurosis has occurred *post* an accident certainly does not prove that it has occurred *propter* the accident . . . one feels, very much to one's embarrassment, that psychiatrists appear to talk of "traumatic" neurosis and "post-traumatic" neurosis virtually as though those two terms were synonymous.'

A look at the current edition of Munkman (1980) on *Damages for Personal Injuries and Death* gives an idea of the compensation rates for injuries. Loss of an arm or a hand comes out at about £10,000–£15,000 and loss of both in the region of £20,000 or more. A severe head injury with post-traumatic epilepsy fetches £40,000–£50,000. But how does one assess 'pain, suffering and inconvenience', especially where the body remains intact? That substantial damages may be awarded for a neurosis was attested in *Liffen* v. *Watson* (1940), in which it was held for a female plaintiff that:

'it was no answer to the claim with respect of neurosis that she could avoid the pain by not doing certain things. The fact that she was prevented by the disease from doing those things was a reason for awarding damages.'

Mr Justice Birkett in *Griffiths* v. *Green & Silley Weir Ltd* (1955), said:

'When people speak of anxiety neurosis when a man is not suffering organically but has hysteria, the ordinary sound, healthy man is apt to look upon that with a little disdain or a little suspicion and to treat it sometimes rather lightly and to say: "Well, if you have a little courage or determination you can overcome it. If you have a little will-power to go back to work and confront the difficulty, that would overcome it." I say it is comparatively easy for healthy people to think and to speak like that, but nobody who has undergone a very severe illness, or indeed a slight illness can forget that people who are not in that happy state frequently look upon small matters as very important.'

In assessing the sum for pain and suffering that judge took the view that neurosis was severe enough to require adequate compensation:

'I can conceive of very few things so painful as to be continually unwell: to lose the savour and zest of life; to be at times afflicted with those violent headaches . . . I think must award a fairly substantial sum on that aspect of the matter.'

Nevertheless, it is a truism that damages for neurosis in post-traumatic situations tend to produce far less in the way of awards than injury to some particular part of the body which is clearly visible, in spite of the fact that the limitations on a patient's life may be more. Although the aim of compensation is to be fair, assessment is clearly difficult in these cases. Mr Justice Pearson, as he then was, in *Tuckey* v. *Green & Silley Weir Ltd* (1955), set out the dilemma:

'The real trouble in assessing damages in this case—I will say it quite frankly, is this: It is very easy to be very wrong either way. If one gives a very large sum, the man may recover in a very short time and go back to face work. On the other hand if one gives a very small sum the man may not recover and will lose a great deal of future wages, and suffer a great deal of pain and suffering, and the sum may be much too small. So in those circumstances one can only do one's best.'

In that assessment for damages must be undertaken at one time and that they are given once and for all, accurate prognosis of the individual case seems vital. As has been indicated in earlier chapters, doctors are often reticent about making predictions in post-traumatic disorders, and studies of follow-up are highly influenced by selection bias of patients. Much has been written, but no adequate studies on morbidity have been undertaken. Doctors make dogmatic statements in court, but the grounds are often shaky. The shakier the ground, the more likely it is that there will be medical opinion acting 'on the other side' stating a contrary opinion.

It goes without saying that there is no dearth of advisers about the legal implications of post-traumatic neurosis, and that almost all the authors quoted in this book have practical advice to offer. Often, of course, the advice depends on whether the writer has the interest of the defendant or the plaintiff in mind and this, of course, has led to a morass of conflict. As was stated earlier, Erichsen's own work was often produced in court after its publication, its presentation only being diminished after the publication of Page's work. Erichsen's own advice to doctors was not to get involved in the amount of compensation payable and, if seeing a patient on behalf of a third party, never to visit the patient beyond the attentions required for the assessment of the accident. He said that no solicitor should be present during examinations and, should the patient's legal adviser insist on being in the room, he felt 'it is better for the examining surgeon to withdraw'. Erichsen, like many others, felt that the situation would be furthered greatly if medical men on both sides were to meet together and confer upon the case to determine a joint report.

'The difference of opinion would probably be found to be narrowed down to one or two points—probably to questions connected with the duration rather than with the nature of the alleged injury.'

Clevenger (1889), while accepting much of what Erichsen said, was more sceptical then Erichsen about the differences that arise between different doctors.

'Such may exist between honest men, but when both sides, as is often the case, do not know what truth is, have become so accustomed to telling lies that they habitually think lies, where can be the "honest difference".... As a rule among regular physicians in consultations where no money issue is at stake, a fair agreement can be reached, but the divergences of opinion in many medico-legal cases are too great to admit of but one conclusion and that is that someone is lying.'

Further studies in the area are clearly required, but also what is needed is more logical understanding of the condition, and a closer collaboration between the medical and legal profession. The final word on litigation aspects should be left to Purves-Stewart (1928) who, highlighting an often overlooked aspect of the whole process, overlooked that it is by the professionals involved, said:

'Litigation neurosis may be likened to an originally innocuous drink to which exciting ingredients are added at the bar—the legal Bar. Such a "cocktail" is expensive, mainly because of its legal ingredients.'

Law Case Reports

Baker *v.* Willoughby (1970) A.C. 467.
Cutler *v.* Vauxhall Motors Ltd (1971) I Q.B. 418.
Griffiths *v.* Green & Silley Weir Ltd (1955) I Lloyds Rep. 190.
James *v.* Woodall Duckham Construction (1969) I W.L.R. 903.
Liffen *v.* Watson (1940) I K.B. 556.
Pearson *v.* Pimms & Sons Ltd 1 26 L.T. 301.
Tuckey *v.* Green & Silley Weir Ltd (1955) 2 Lloyds Rep. 619.

References

Bebbington, P. (1980) Causal models and logical inference in epidemiological psychiatry. *British Journal of Psychiatry* **136**, 317.

Brend, W. A. (1938) *Traumatic Mental Disorders in Courts of Law.* William Heinemann, London.

Clevenger, S. V. (1889) *Spinal Concussion.* F. A. Davis, London.

Collie, J. (1933) *Workman's Compensation, its Medical Aspect.* Edward Arnold and Co., London.

Ellard, J. (1970) Psychological reactions to compensable injury. *Medical Journal of Australia* **2**, 349.

Jolowicz, J. A., Lewis, T. E. and Harris, D. M. (1971) *Winfield and Jolowicz on Tort.* 9th Edition. Sweet and Maxwell, London.

Kalinowsky, L. B. (1950) Problems of war neuroses in light of experiences in other countries. *American Journal of Psychiatry* **107**, 340.

Kräupl Taylor, F. (1979) *The Concepts of Illness, Disease and Morbus.* Cambridge University Press, London.

Lewy, E. (1941) Compensation for war neurosis. *War Medicine* **1**, 887.

Munkman, J. (1980) *Damages for Personal Injuries and Death.* 6th Edition. Butterworths, London.

Ogus, A. I. (1973) *The Law of Damages.* Butterworths, London.

Purves-Stewart, J. (1928) Discussion on traumatic neurasthenia and litigation neurosis. *Proceedings of the Royal Society of Medicine* **21**, 359.

Slater, J. K. (1946) Trauma and the nervous system. *Edinburgh Medical Journal* **53**, 623.

CHAPTER 9

Conclusion

The ideas surrounding post-traumatic neurosis and related problems reviewed in this text, like so many in medicine, seem to reflect those prevalent at any particular time in history. Thus in the nineteenth century there was an emphasis on the organic material changes that occurred following an accident, with a search for the 'organic cause'. This was followed by a period of psychological interpretation of the symptoms, hinted at by Charcot and synthesized by Freud and his followers, at a time in history when there was a 'Romantic rebound' from earlier materialism. Finally, the last 20 years has seen again some reversal in trend, some reaction to this early century Romanticism, with a current emphasis once more on the 'organic'. There have at all times, of course, been supporters of the alternative view to the predominant one ready to express their position, and mention has been made of these. What makes one view favoured at any particular time is difficult to determine, but presumably reflects the readiness of a particular society to accept, read about, talk about, and generally uphold the position, rather than cold objective logic. It would not be amiss to suggest that, where opinion fluctuates from one pole to another, the answer to the problem is perhaps to be sought at some midway point. Far from being an indeterminate 'fence-sitting', this provides a logical way out of an otherwise insoluble position, as long as the evidence presented fits the hypothesis. Before discussing more fully the possibilities of a synthesis of the views on post-traumatic neurosis, with hopefully greater understanding, it is germane to discuss in brief the two sides of the debate expressed at various points in this book so far.

Initially it must be said that for a clinical problem as prevalent as post-traumatic neurosis, affecting thousands of people and costing governments, insurance companies, and others millions of pounds, relatively few studies have been conducted. Often those that have been carried out have been done on highly selected patients, in very special situations. Thus Miller's patients were all cases referred by insurance companies; Merskey's patients often referred by prosecuting solicitors; Symonds' patients were all Forces' personnel. Many writers have confused opinion with fact, and in particular have neglected findings contradictory to their own ideas. Pejorative, rather than scientific, expression has been used in discussing patients with post-traumatic problems, and the 'anti-scientific' mistrust of academic excellence in the courtroom has been alluded to.

The earlier studies on post-traumatic sequelae tended to dwell on losses of bodily parts and, in the case of nervous symptoms, tended to ascribe them to organic causes. The views of Erichsen and others, such as Brodie, were typical of this era, but the majority of their ideas were based on opinion, and they produced little other than anecdotes to support their claims. Nevertheless, they did serve to highlight a clinical problem, and raised the possibility that post-traumatic neurotic symptoms, especially if consequent to brain or spinal cord damage, may have their origins in organic changes. These were often seen in terms of functional, as opposed to structural change, and their views received support from contemporary neuropathologists.

By the end of the nineteenth century, with the writings of such authors as Page and Charcot, ideas were altering to accept 'psychic' factors in the aetiology of neurotic symptoms, and the concept of 'nervous shock' became accepted in the literature. Although seemingly the idea was straightforward, the actual mechanism whereby clinical change occurred was not formulated, until writers of the Freudian and post-Freudian eras embarked on their psychoanalytical interpretations. With such psychological explanations for health, illness, and personality structure, and with the considerable growth of psychiatry as an independent discipline, especially in the United States of America, the association of psychological theorizing with psychiatry was commonplace, and dissociation between psychiatry and neurology became complete. 'Psychological' developed several different meanings. Initially the Freudian model implied some internal structure to the mind which, on account of conflict and trauma, underwent reorganization to produce symptoms. 'Psychogenic' implied a mechanism which, originally at least, had some relationship with the brain. However, it gradually lost such associations, and eventually became equated with 'psychosocial', with the implication that disorders were due to external causes related to the person's environment.

In spite of the fact that most psychoanalytical speculation has never been tested in any scientific way, the hold such ideas had, and still have, over the thinking and theorizing of many people has led to a clouding of psychiatric concepts, and a misunderstanding of problems such as post-traumatic neurosis. One effect of the separation between neurology and psychiatry has been the insistence that disorders were either psychological or organic in origin, and the concept of an interaction became lost. The brain and the mind were divorced. Organic disorders were clearly understood as disorders related to neurological disease of the brain, and where such disease could not be demonstrated, the problem was called functional, which term lost its original meaning and became synonymous with psychological. Finally, in relation to post-traumatic neurosis in particular, 'functional' became used pejoratively, in the eyes of many being equated with malingering, putting it on and play-acting. Patients who developed neurotic symptoms after injury were required to have clearly defined organic injuries, and neurological signs accompanying them, in order to be considered 'genuine', and if such evidence was lacking they were regarded as malingerers. However, those who espoused such views were usually guilty of the same mistakes made by others before them. They put forward opinion, and failed to present any refutable facts. Among those who attempted to provide some figures was Collie (1917), whose evidence indicated that illness following injury seemed susceptible to manipulation by compensation factors, although it is clear that he really thought that most people were not acting out of malice. Our mind, he commented, runs along the lines of least resistance; society, he suggested, makes the conditions ripe for post-traumatic neurosis to develop. Kamman (1951) too avoided the malingering issue by the suggestion that the abnormal attitudes developing in the face of a compensation are part of a personality disorder rather than overt malicious fraud. However, none of these ideas helped decide who was, and who was not, out to defraud for his own personal gain, and who should be considered ill and in need of medical help and deserve compensation.

A main difficulty is that clear clinical differences have not been demonstrated between patients regarded as malingering, and patients regarded as having a neurosis. From the literature, however, several guidelines emerge. First, the studies carried out in the war setting with attempts to assess premorbid personality traits and to quantify 'stress', led to the acknowledgement of the 'neurotic constitution', and gave clues how to recognize it in a clinical examination. Some patients, by virtue of their neurotic character, are more prone to break down under stress than others. In addition, those who attempted to grade stress indicated that its severity interacted with the underlying personality in a quantitative way. Minimal stress will precipitate breakdown in patients with severe premorbid neuroticism, whereas maximal stress will be required in patients with good premorbid personalities. However, everyone has a breaking point and will break down under severe stress. The situation of sudden disaster, representing extreme stress, is seen in this light, precipitating illness readily in those predisposed, but also in many without apparent constitutional liability. The negative results of some studies in the assessment of the constitutional factor in determining neurotic illness may be due to an inadequate collection of the personal history data of patients, with a neglect of pre-existing factors indicative of neuroticism. In any case, the number of studies highlighting the relationship to predisposition are in excess of those with negative findings.

The type of breakdown encountered may be of a classical hysteria with paralyses or similar presentations, or may be the type of neurosis which presents with symptoms of anxiety and depression with associated complaints such as palpitations, sleeplessness, panic attacks, breathlessness, and phobias. The presence of these symptoms in particular, whether or not associated with apparent physical illness, would be in favour of a diagnosis of neurosis, and renders malingering doubtful. Why certain patients develop one pattern of illness, and not another, is unknown. Predisposition to develop certain types of symptoms may be constitutional, dependent on genetic and epigenetic factors. There is substantial evidence to show that affective illness has a genetic basis, and the same may be said for the neuroses (see Slater and Roth, 1960). Some personality types may be more prone to develop hysterical phenomena than others. Kretschmer (1948), who had considerable experience with hysterical phenomena in the war setting, denied the existence of any 'hysterical type'. He felt that 'a pre-disposition towards hysterical reactions is widespread and, in the last analysis, deeply rooted in the instinctive mechanism common to all men'. Others have more clearly defined the 'hysterical personality' as patients who have egocentric attitudes, tend to enjoy exhibitionism and dramatism, are emotionally shallow, but are excitable with affective lability, are dependent, suggestible, flirtatious but frigid, in speech employ verbal exaggeration, and are impulsive in decision-making. (For review see Trimble, 1981.) Such a personality type has been strongly associated with hysterical symptoms, although the available studies do not entirely support this conclusion. Ljungberg (1957) for example, in a study of 381 patients with conversion phenomena, found 43% of males and 47% of women to have deviant personalities, but only 21% of the total conformed to the hysterical type. Merskey and Trimble (1979), in a study of 89 patients with hysteria, noted 17 with hysterical personalities, and while this was a higher frequency than in a control population with psychiatric illness, clearly other personality types were represented in the hysteria population.

Malingering must of course remain a possible diagnosis in some patients, but how is it recognized? The most persuasive arguments for malingering, such as those made by Miller, hardly give clear guidelines for its detection. Malingering is, after all, a diagnosis in the same way that depression and multiple sclerosis are diagnoses, and criteria must be specified for its recognition. Hurst, in his book did give some positive guidelines which would seem useful, although in practice usually a diagnosis of malingering is implied without positive evidence. To make a diagnosis on purely negative grounds may do a great injustice to patients, and is not good medical practice. Miller's own results were based on patients mainly referred by insurance companies, and other follow-up studies after compensation has been settled do not lead to his conclusions, indicating residual morbidity in a high percentage of cases.

There is in fact absence of hard evidence to support the contention that most patients with post-traumatic neurosis are malingering, which has to be weighed against the evidence now accumulating to demonstrate that, at least after head injuries, organic change may occur within the central nervous system, and be responsible in some cases for the ensuing symptomatology. Thus the animal experiments discussed in Chapter 5 provide data on observed physiological changes that occur with head injury, and the physical explanations of Holbourn, borne out by the studies of Pudenz and Sheldon, provide an explanation of the mechanism of contre-coup injuries, and in particular of damage to the frontal and temporal lobes of the brain that can occur after impact. The neuropathological data pinpoint subtle neuronal damage that occurs even after relatively trivial injury, providing backing for the warnings of the animal experimenters that '... some cell loss will occur in all concussions ...' (Groat and Simmons, 1950).

Clinically, however, even if some form of neuronal loss does occur with accidents, it is still not clear how it can be detected and how it influences subsequent behaviour. On the first point, the absence of clearly defined organic changes detected on clinical neurological and psychological examination is frequently quoted as implying that no organic changes have occurred. However, if it is remembered that clinical neurological examination and standard psychometric testing assess changes in those parts of the brain that subserve motor, sensory, and cognitive abilities, in particular cortical deficits, it is of no surprise that, without more sophisticated techniques, organic changes, if present, remain undetected. The regions of the brain primarily affected by closed head injuries seem to be the midbrain, temporal and frontal cortex, and areas in and around the limbic system. Lesions in these sites lead not to clear isolated deficits of activity, with for example paralysis of a group of muscles, but rather to changes in behaviour, mood, and feeling. The disturbed behaviour itself, in particular the neuroses, may therefore be a reflection of underlying neuronal damage. It is clear from the studies reviewed, however, that to date such a hypothesis has not been clearly formulated, or experimentally tested. One possible reason for this is that only recently has it been possible, with a rapid increase in our knowledge of neurochemistry and the exploration experimentally of brain–behaviour relationships, to synthesize a psychobiological view of human activity, and once again explain functional disorders more precisely in terms of disturbed brain function.

Thus it will be recalled that originally the term 'functional disorder', used in association with the concept of organic disorder, implied disease attributed to altered function, rather than structure, of neuronal processes.

Charcot, and to some extent Freud especially in his earlier years, were implying that subtle changes in neuronal activity occurred to account for functional disorders. Freud (1948) for example stated:

'I will take the word functional or dynamic lesion in its proper sense: "alteration in function of mechanism". Such an alteration, for example, would be a diminution in excitability or in a physiological quality which in the normal state remains constant or varies within fixed limits. . . .'

The later developments of the psychoanalytic writers and the degradation of the concept of functional disorders has been outlined. Throughout this century, however, there have been attempts to support the concept that functional disorders have some biologically defined basis, and the writings of Kinear Wilson and Foster-Kennedy have already been mentioned. Others who have maintained this tradition include Symonds (1926), Schilder (1940), Slater (1943), Cobb (1944), Stengel (1949), and Lewis (1971).

A turning point in the history of psychiatry, still ignored by many, was the description in the 1920s of encephalitis lethargica and its consequences by von Economo (1931). Following certain influenza epidemics it was observed that a number of patients developed a wide range of behavioural abnormalities from hyperkinesis to Parkinsonism, to personality changes and frank psychiatric illness. The pathological changes that occurred were seen primarily in the midbrain and brain-stem. Von Economo stated:

'Hardly ever has the discovery of a disease not only taught us so many separate new facts, but altered our outlook so radically; . . . just as we find it hard today to follow up the trend of thought of our scientific predecessors for whom bacteriology and the love of brain localisation did not exist, future scientific generations will hardly be able to appreciate our pre-encephalitic neurological and psychiatric conceptions, particularly with regard to so-called functional disturbance. To emphasise the difference of encephalitis lethargica from most of the nervous diseases known till the present day, it must be remembered that the majority of the latter are system diseases, . . . with injury to the long tracts and their continuations and the association-tracts. All conditions other than those diseases were generally looked upon as functional disorders. . . . Now we can, in a similar manner, describe encephalitis lethargica as a functional affection, but on an organic basis . . . our disease . . . proves the essential role which quite a number of anatomical structures play with regard to our psychological processes and their arrangements.'

Amongst the symptoms described by von Economo, as a consequence of the disease, were disturbances of volition or 'will', so neatly separated by dualists from the general consideration of somatic processes. Symonds (1926) pointed out the similarity of the mental symptoms which resulted from toxaemia, encephalitis lethargica, and 'undigested worry', and Schilder (1940) further developed the theme that the same symptoms could develop from either psychological or organic disturbance. He stated: 'Cerebral organic syndromes may change functions of the brain in such a way as to provoke neurotic attitudes. . . .' Stengel (1949) made the point:

'Often a neurotic syndrome forms round a nucleus of symptoms due to structural damage, especially when the latter is slight. It is difficult and unprofitable to attempt to demarcate the neurotic superstructure from what is called its organic basis. . . .'

Such comments have been borne out experimentally in studies on patients presenting with hysteria. Thus many are reported to have structural cerebral disorders (Whitlock, 1967; Merskey and Buhrich, 1975), and the interactional aspects of these with other factors, in the production of the clinical syndrome, has been emphasized (Merskey and Trimble, 1979).

What, however, are the functional changes? Originally functional disorders were distinguished from structural disorders on the grounds that patients with the latter had observable changes after death. This idea was seen to be fallacious by von Economo among others, as clearly it depended primarily on the power of the methods used to detect changes. With modern techniques and knowledge the line between functional and organic becomes very blurred. Thus if changes not visible by simple microscopy are seen on the electron microscope they may be related to altered function, but are still presumably alterations of structure. Jelliffe (1933) avoided this dilemma by commenting:

'I talk of "reversible" and "irreversible" organic changes, never of organic changes. Organic changes are always taking place in all functioning organs. Anyone should know that, whether within the physiological range, or whether reversible or not is the important consideration.'

It is clear that if the term functional is to have any useful meaning in the neurosciences it must refer to disordered functioning within the nervous system. Any abnormality which leads to alteration of a person's behaviour, which may be detected clinically, may be the result of structural lesions, but also may occur in their absence, especially if it is primarily a change of neurotransmitter or receptor activity. Disturbed function may be expressed neurologically, as a paralysis for example, or psychiatrically as a neurosis or psychosis. In neurological practice the structural lesion is sought, and the clinical examination is used to localize the site of the offending lesion. In psychiatric practice this is not done, usually because psychiatric signs and symptoms defy simple localization. In fact the equation of function with 'activity', and the implication that altered activity following a structural lesion suggested the function of the part of the brain destroyed, has been quite misleading in neurology (Blake Pritchard, 1955; Riese, 1950). As Hughlings Jackson and others have pointed out, it may be possible to localize a lesion but not a function.

'Symptoms, lesions, and functional systems are not comparable, cannot be, as it were, superimposed one on the other, and obey differing rules of localisation.' (Wilson, 1930)

One mechanism whereby patients develop psychiatric illness following accident or threat has already been discussed. Thus constitutional liability, combined with trauma, can lead to the production of symptoms. There is substantial evidence in the psychiatric literature which shows that life events lead to the precipitation of illness, and accidents of the type discussed must be considered as significant life events. Thus the occurrence of events, especially stressful events, is associated with a 2–6 fold increase in the risk for depression and other neurotic illness over the ensuing six months. Such events are seen as interacting with personality and previous experience to result in symptoms (Paykel, 1978). However, many people develop symptoms without clear evidence of such a neurotic personality, and the evidence reviewed here suggests that this is a common event after a head injury. If, as suggested, the same symptoms can result from psychologically induced and organically induced disturbance, the mechanism of the behaviour changes following head injury in some of these cases becomes clear. The evidence suggests that small structural lesions occur in the midbrain and diencephalon in head injuries, and the possibility of similar subtle changes in the limbic system has also been raised. As Stengel (1949) commented: 'Neurotic symptoms are apt to emerge . . . whenever the resources of the personality have suffered through injury to the brain.' The reason is that the 'resistance of the personality, and its ability to deal with the impact of environmental stress, have suffered'. The patient becomes, as it were, prone to the development of the neuroses, in the same way that someone with constitutional neurotic traits is susceptible. This view receives substantial support from the work of Slater (1943) who stated:

'Organic and neurotic symptoms will be clinically indistinguishable one from another. Further, the organic injury may itself predispose to neurosis, which will occur in its presence with a lesser intensity of constitutional instability than otherwise necessary.'

The precise mechanism of symptom production by such damage remains to be elucidated, but the same result it seems can arise from lesions situated at different sites within the central nervous system. Psychic processes cannot be strictly localized, and as such represent the outcome of integrative action of the central nervous system. It is here suggested that damage to some regions of the brain, in particular the limbic system and its connections, is more liable to induce neurosis than damage to others, although all lesions, however small, may undermine the individual's ability to manipulate his environment successfully, and result in or exacerbate a neurosis.

At some time in the future it may be possible to explain further, at a more precise neurophysiological level, how changes in behaviour come about. Recent advances in this direction include attempts to observe changes in brain biochemistry in psychiatric illness. In the 1950s, with the development of the electron microscope, the old argument over whether or not the neurones represented a reticular mass of connected tissue or were separate entities, was finally settled, with the delineation of the structure of neurones and the synaptic cleft. Neurotransmitters, identified earlier in peripheral nerves, were seen within the central nervous system, and techniques for delineating various neurotransmitter pathways were described. The monoamine systems in particular assumed great importance, since it seemed that clearly identifiable tracts for each of several substances existed, and that for many, the cells of origin were in the brain-stem and midbrain. From these regions axons travelled to areas in the hypothalamus, limbic and striatal areas, and thence to the cortex, such that one cell of origin would make synaptic connections with many thousands of other neurones (see Figure 9.1). The possibility that damage to such systems could thus have far reaching consequences for an individual's behaviour is obvious, an idea supported by observations that drugs which depleted these systems of their neurotransmitters lead to a behavioural state of depression, and that many psychotropic drugs, introduced for the management of depression, tend to increase the availability of these monoamines within the synaptic cleft. Alterations of the metabolism of a variety of substances, including monoamines have been described after head injury (Hyyppa *et al.*, 1977), and provide an important link between the organic structural and the functional aspects of post-traumatic illness.

The results of the psychologists who have investigated these problems, discussed in Chapter 5, have indicated that disturbed performance, especially on tasks requiring sustained attention, occurs in patients with post-traumatic symptoms. Conventional psychological testing is often normal, however, and the reasons for this are clear. They are primarily concerned with assessing higher cortical function, and tests used were designed to isolate and identify localized cortical lesions. The tests are time-based, and as such do not give information

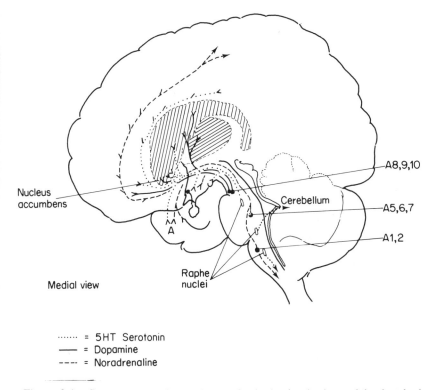

Figure 9.1   Some monoamine pathways in the brain. A, Amygdala; hatched area, caudate nucleus/putamen (from Trimble 1981)

about how individuals are impaired on continuous tasks. But living is a sustained task, and it is perhaps no coincidence that many post-traumatic neurotic symptoms occur when patients attempt to return to work. If their performance is impaired, as some psychological test results suggest, then it is not surprising that they fail to cope with a job that previously they had coped with quite well. Their capacity to receive and deal with information from the environment is diminished, and overload of their ability occurs at a lower level than previously, such that soon fatiguability and concentration difficulties develop.

There are then at least two possible and compatible explanations for the development of neurotic symptoms following injury. The first is related to the neurotic constitution and liability to breakdown under stress; the other is based on neuropathology subsequent to head injury. It is suggested that there is some experimental evidence to support these ideas, and little or no evidence to support a hypothesis that all or even most such patients are malingering. In many, a combination of both constitutional liability and minimal brain damage may provide the resulting picture. Not all patients, however, fall into such easy groupings as this, and for others alternative explanations need to be invoked. Doubtless in some patients the psychoanalytical interpretation, based on symbolism and unresolved conflicts, is an appropriate one, but to date has proved resistant to experimental verification. Lishman (1978) demonstrated with a case history some of the difficulties involved in assessment, and in particular the impossibility of attaining a full understanding of the aetiology of the patient's symptoms at one brief interview:

'A woman of 45 was disabled for many months by a number of neurotic complaints after surviving intact from a car crash. The head injury had been mild but her vision had been threatened for a time. Her persistent neurotic reaction was surprising in view of her excellent previous mental health and stability. She eventually confessed to a longstanding secret liaison with the husband of a friend, in whose company the accident had occurred.'

He suggested that the injury served as a focus for longstanding guilt and continuing emotional distress.

Certainly some of these ideas help explain the pattern of some symptoms, especially in hysteria, although other possibilities were put forward by Charcot. Still another suggestion came from Huddleston (1932):

'A previous injury, illness or neurotic disability, with localisation in the back for example, can have created a locus minoris resistantiae so that a camptocormia may follow another injury as readily as one to the skull or spine. . . . The symptoms of a previous head injury now healed are frequently perpetuated in the neurosis.'

Other patients who may be prone to develop post-traumatic neurosis, even in the absence of organic injury, may include those who are obsessional and controlling of their environment, and who find being out of control at the time of the accident quite overwhelming, and those that have been so protected throughout their life that they are particularly prone to develop a neurosis when they finally face danger, since they do not, as it were, build up an appropriate immunity to life's stresses. These suggestions, however, remain as speculations, open to verification.

It is hoped that some light has been thrown on possible mechanisms involved in the production of post-traumatic syndromes, and in particular post-traumatic neurosis. What is clear is that generalization about these problems is naïve, especially with our relative lack of information, and to suppose the problem is all one thing, or another does injustice to individual patients. It is suggested that for many patients seen in practice the adage still is appropriate:

The patient says he cannot
The staff say he will not
The truth is, the patient cannot will.

References

Blake Pritchard, E. A. (1955) The functional symptoms of organic disease of the brain. *Lancet* i, 363.
Cobb, S. (1944) *Foundations of Neuropsychiatry*. Williams and Wilkins, Baltimore.
Collie, J. (1917) *Malingering and Feigned Sickness*. Edward Arnold, London.
Freud, S. (1948) Some points in a comparative study of organic and hysterical paralysis. *Collected Papers I*. Hogarth Press, London.
Groat, R. A. and Simmons, J. Q. (1950) Loss of nerve cells in experimental cerebral concussion. *Journal of Neuropathology and Experimental Neurology* 9, 150.
Huddleston, J. H. (1932) *Accidents, Neuroses and Compensation*. Williams and Wilkins, Baltimore.
Hyyppa, M. T., Långuik, V., Nieminen, V. and Vapalahti, M. (1977) Tryptophan and monoamine metabolites in ventricular cerebrospinal fluid after severe cerebral trauma. *Lancet* 11, 1367.
Jelliffe, S. E. (1933) *Reply to book Review*. Archives of Neurology and Psychiatry 30, 239.
Kamman, G. R. (1951) Traumatic neurosis, compensation neurosis or attitude pathosis? *Archives of Neurology and Psychiatry* 65, 593.
Kretschmer, E. (1948) *Hysteria, Reflex and Instinct* (1961). Peter Owen, London.
Lewis, A. (1971) 'Endogenous' and 'exogenous': a useful dichotomy. *Psychological Medicine* 1, 191.
Lishman, W. A. (1978) *Organic Psychiatry*. Blackwells, London.
Ljungberg, L. (1957) Hysteria. *Acta Psychiatrica Scandinavica* Suppl. 112.
Merskey, H. and Buhrich, N. A. (1975) Hysteria and organic brain disease. *British Journal of Medical Psychology* 48, 359.
Merskey, H. and Trimble, M. R. (1979) Personality, sexual adjustment and

brain lesions in patients with conversion symptoms. *American Journal of Psychiatry* **136**, 179.

Paykel, E. S. (1978) Contribution of life events to causation of psychiatric illness. *Psychological Medicine* **8**, 245.

Riese, W. (1950) *Principles of Neurology.* Nervous and Mental Disease Monographs, New York.

Schilder, P. (1940) Neuroses following head and brain injuries. In *Injuries of the Skull, Brain and Spinal Cord.* Ed. Brock, S. Williams and Wilkins, Philadelphia.

Slater, E. (1943) The neurotic constitution. *Journal of Neurology and Psychiatry* **6**, 1.

Slater, E. and Roth, M. (1960) *Clinical Psychiatry.* Baillière Tindall and Cassell, London.

Stengel, E. (1949) Borderlands of neurology and psychiatry. In *Recent Progress in Psychiatry* **11**, 1.

Symonds, C. P. (1926) Functional or organic? Some points of view. *Lancet* **i**, 64.

Trimble, M. R. (1981) *Neuropsychiatry.* J. Wiley and Sons, Chichester.

Von Economo, C. (1931) *Encephalitis Lethargica. Its sequelae and treatment.* Trans. Newman, K. O. Oxford University Press, London.

Whitlock, F. A. (1967) The aetiology of hysteria. *Acta Psychiatrica Scandinavica* **43**, 144.

Wilson, S. A. K. (1930) Nervous semeiology with special reference to epilepsy. *British Medical Journal* **2**, 1.

Index